Fire In The Belly

The Surprise Cause Of Most Diseases, Mental States and Aging Processes

By Keith Scott-Mumby MD, MB ChB, PhD

Published by Mother Whale Inc.

PO Box 19452, Reno, Nevada, 89511, USA

Cover design and layout by Dragos Balasoiu (www.bold-pixel.com)

Disclaimer

Contents

part 2 Quenching The Flames

Introduction

The Biggest Medical Revolution Ever?

This book describes what is certainly one of the most far-reaching and profound shifts in scientific medical opinion since the development of the germ theory of infectious diseases. It engenders a whole new way of looking at how disease comes about, how genes work and the importance of inflammation in our defences and in the process of aging.

If that's not enough, it's also about having a whole second brain in the guts, something so shocking and surprising, that most doctors and scientists are still reeling from its implications.

In the 1970s and 80s I stood at the threshold of this gateway, with a handful of other doctors around the world (less than a dozen of us, full time). We got results—fabulous recoveries, miracles even—without fully understanding what we were seeing. For pioneer spirits and for doctors looking for real healing, that didn't worry us too much. We knew the methods worked and that sooner or later the science would be figured out.

Even so, the final answer, now it is in view, is so far removed from what we imagined, I must say that even I am shocked by these new revelations.

It might seem from the title that I will be talking about colitis, celiac disease, Crohn's disease, irritable bowel, and so on. This is wrong! I shall be talking about whole body disease, from migraines and asthma, to arthritis and autoimmune diseases, to behavior disorders and chronic depression. In fact I should repeat: this is about the way almost all diseases originate or are impacted by what goes on in the intestines.

It may even be about why we have sex!

The modern view of biological evolution is what has been christened "The Red Queen scenario"; it replaced an older model called the "tangled bank". The Red Queen (from the Alice In Wonderland books) had to run and run and run, just to stay in the same place.

In evolution, we have to change and change and change, otherwise the pathogens will nail us. We change, new barriers; they evolve a new strategy, so we change again and the pathogens evolve yet another strategy of attack. Neither side is winning; healthy people are just changing fast enough to stay ahead. But like the Red Queen, we must run and run and run.

Scientists speculate this is why sex came about. After all, reproduction is easy: we just divide in two, right? But we don't do it that way; we swap genes, which needs sex and transmission of seed chromosomes to egg chromosomes. Re-mixing genes in this way is like spinning the lock on a combination safe. We lock out the pathogens.

But pretty soon they figure out the new combination and they are back in. But because we have sex and keep changing our gene combination, we mostly stay healthy. BUT THAT'S HOW BIG A DEAL THIS IS!

It's virtually a host-pathogen arms race!

The Friendly Fifth Column

But it's even more subtle than that. We are host to an army of micro-organisms (microbes) that is fighting on our side. Without this army, we could never hope to defeat the many pathogens that consider us humans a legitimate target.

They are like a fifth column of insiders, that relay information about "the enemy" and help us keep our weapons in order. We know just how important this is from what happens when we destroy our fifth column: overuse of antibiotics has damaged and rendered this friendly army inside us ineffective in some individuals and they get very sick—even die as a result.

This book is largely about understanding and working with our friendly army, so that we can enjoy the best of health, using the best of science.

Make no mistake, if you don't pay attention, you'll sicken fast, age before you need to and die relatively young. Chronically sick people do not live until extreme old age. Only pretty healthy people make it to their 90s and beyond.

The "army" we call the human microbiota. You know how scientists like fancy names. Microbiota just means little organisms. I'll be showing you how this includes bacteria, viruses (an amazing lot of those!), parasites, molds, yeasts, protozoa and other funny little critters.

But their effect is not so little. Indeed, it is emerging that they are the main reason we are healthy or sick. I became internationally-known in the 1980s and 90s for my work with food allergies: telling people what they should and shouldn't eat, to enjoy optimum health. Food "allergy" was just a convenience word; most of these reactions had no classic signs of an allergic mechanism.

But there was no doubt about the amazing recoveries. What I understand now is that doctors like me were tuning the diet to keep the patient's microbiota happy and flourishing; or if it had been damaged by poor nutrition, debility or antibiotics, we brought it back to strength and vitality.

I've always argued it was arrogant of doctors to think they cured disease; it's Nature who cures, the wise physician merely sets the stage. But never in my wildest dreams did I realize the extent to which this critical army of tiny soldiers were actually doing the work.

By helping and cherishing the infantry soldiers down there in the gut, we were able to effect miracles. It's very humbling, looking back. We fixed autism, ADD, eczema, asthma, arthritis, schizophrenia, colitis, IBS, ulcers, MS and a whole host of diverse conditions and I felt very privileged as a doctor. For the first time in my working life I really cured people—and I used that term advisedly—and now I understand how much of it was done, it's even more awesome to contemplate!

That Second Brain

Earlier I mentioned a "second brain" in the guts. You probably thought that was just a metaphor. But it's not. We do have a virtual brain in our intestines.

There is a vast neural network that is many ways rivals the brain in the skull. It's called the enteric nervous system, or ENS (as opposed to the central nervous system, or CNS). There are more neurons in the gut (over 100 million) than in the spinal cord.

There's all the usual synaptic, electrical and chemical buzz going on in our guts, same as in the brain. It's remarkable.

Traditionally, the nervous system has been divided into the voluntary (conscious) nervous system and the autonomic nervous system (sympathetic and parasympathetic). Now it's clear that we need to add the third element, the ENS.

Thing is, the ENS has all the neurotransmitters of the upper brain: there's serotonin (5-HT) down there, in fact 90% of the body's serotonin is in the gut! That's our "happy" neurotransmitter. Unfortunately, serotonin is also pro-inflammatory (causes inflammation).

But there's also acetyl choline, noradrenaline or norepinephrine as the Americans call it, glutamine, gamma-aminobutyric acid and encephalins, plus endorphins and weird stuff you don't need to know about, such as cocaine-and-amphetamine-regulated-transcript (CART). I'm looking at a list of 28 on my desk!

So the idea of a second brain in the guts suddenly doesn't seem so crazy, does it? That explains the nice happy feeling after a good feed; why we feel calm and sleepy after Christmas pudding and a glass of port; and why being in a sour mood spoils our digestion!

Does this matter? You bet! Take as an example the case of what we used to call "leaky gut syndrome". It's a bit difficult to nail down but a simple enough concept: over the years, the gut wall gets damaged and starts to "leak" or allow through larger molecules than are needed or are healthy. See, if the molecules are big enough, they are capable of setting up an allergic reaction. Hence food allergy and intolerance.

All very nice. But the missing ingredient here is that the bowel naturally has what are called "tight junctions" between the cells and they do not leak. It's the enteric nervous system that serves as a gate and can open and shut these tight junctions in just moments (like sluice gates to a dam). So it's not damage over the years, at all, that makes the gut leak. It's an unhappy gut brain!

Wow. We need to keep our guts happy. That means not eating the wrong foods and that's why the "Scott-Mumby Diet" and other low-allergy plans work so well. Inflammatory foods are deadly, because they blast open the gates of these tight junctions and start the mayhem of systemic (total body) inflammation.

Microbiota, Mood and Behavior

So if there is a gut brain and foods affect it, then foods affect mood. That's obviously true. Now we know why.

In fact there is a continuous cross-talk between our microbiome and our brains. It has emerged that significant stress can produce dysbiosis, as it's called, within hours. That means a major shift in balance of the gut microbiome, in response to mood and emotion, happening very quickly indeed. Much faster than we ever imagined.

It also considerably modifies our view of what people describe as "Candida" and yeasts. Although the condition exists, I've never been as fan of the "Candida" explanation, as fans of my earlier books will realize. Now I realize that this model of supposed dysbiosis is actually wide of the mark. Mood-brain-microbiome disorder (MBMD to go American) would be a better term, or at least more accurate, but I'm not seriously suggesting it.

I am reminded of Len McEwen's PIMS, which he described in the 1980s. It stands for psychology-irritable bowel-migraine syndrome and well describes the relationship between gut symptoms, mood and physical distress.

Dr. Natasha Campbell-McBride seems to have purloined the idea with her GAPS (gut and psychology syndrome). Like most Americans, she's pretty bad at acknowledging those who have gone before her.

The important point is that it's a two-way traffic. As well as mood affecting the microbiome, the microbiome affects mood. In fact anxiety and depression levels can be raised quickly, just by inoculating new bugs.

Not Just The Gut

Finally, it needs pointing out that these important new principles do not only apply to intestinal health. Our microbiome spreads through out our bodies and surface skin, as you will read. To put some numbers to the profusion of our companion "army", let's say this:

- Skin – 1012 (one trillion) resident bacteria
- Mouth – 1010 (ten billion)
- Gut – 1014 (one hundred trillion) mainly in the distal portion
- The total weight approximately 2 – 5 lbs.
- There are about 500 – 1,000 different species
- 99% of the population is made up of 30- 40 main species; predominantly just two: bacteroides and firmiculites.

By contrast we have just maybe 10 trillion body cells, so we are seriously outnumbered!

I have talked about just the "microbiome" but really there is a gut microbiome, skin microbiome, vaginal microbiome etc. These can be further subdivided.

Now for the really scary thing: these microbes together encode up to about 10 million unique genes between them. Humans have only about 25,000 genes, give or take. That means were are out-gunned with genes to a factor of hundreds.

These genes affect the way our body obtains and uses nutrients, detoxes chemicals, deals with food, breaks down polysaccharides, metabolizes hormones and scores of other functions.

There, you missed it, didn't you? I just described the most amazing medical/biological discovery of all time; the one that is so stunning it's hard to believe! What is it? Read the next part of this sentence slowly and carefully: bacterial and other microbial genes from our guts tell our bodies what to do, just like human genes do.

That's remarkable. It is counter-intuitive and doesn't seem right, in the natural order of things. You would think only human genes can tell a human body how to behave. But it just ain't so; so get used to it. Our little troop of hangers on and assistants have as much control over our bodies as our own tissues do (maybe more!)

We are a crowd; a collective, that has been described as "Planet Human", with trillions of inhabitants. You're just one of them!

There are many other shocks and surprises like this on the way, as you work through this text. Enjoy the exciting new discoveries. Make sure you understand them, because the implications are unimaginably far-reaching. It changes the whole science of health and medicine.

There are many sections to the book, building up into the full picture. You need to have all parts of the jigsaw, to see the true puzzle revealed.

I have divided the book into aspects, starting with the clinical manifestations and the many causes.

Enjoy!

This book should be read in conjunction with my Parasites Handbook… and Diet Wise, the best possible self-help book in telling you what to do about this.

part 1

What's On Fire?

Chapter 1 Our Bodies Are Ablaze!

Our bellies are ablaze! Seriously! There is so much inflammatory fire in the human gut that it could be said to be origin of almost all disease. Hippocrates thought so; "All diseases begin in the gut," he said.

Not just bodily diseases but diseases of the mind too. French psychiatrist Phillipe Pinel (1745- 1826, known as the father of modern psychiatry) stated, "The primary seat of insanity is the region of the stomach and intestines."

When you have read more of this book, you will come to understand just how accurate these strange sounding assessments really were.

The inflammatory processes going on in the stomach and bowel are enough to disturb the entire physiological set up of the brain and body, resulting in a plethora of symptoms and complaints—many trivial and inconvenient, to be sure—but some conditions dangerous and even life-threatening.

"But my guts don't give me any problem," you might say.

"But my guts don't give me any problem," you might say. Not true. You may be unaware of symptoms arising *directly* from the intestines but, over the last forty years as a top expert in food intolerance, allergies and dysbiosis, I have found almost every disease imaginable has some connection with the bowel and digestion.

If digestive malfunction isn't the actual *cause* of the complaint, then inflammatory overload due to foods and gut flora certainly aggravate the problem and need to be eliminated, to get a lasting cure.

It's that important. Hippocrates and Pinel were right!

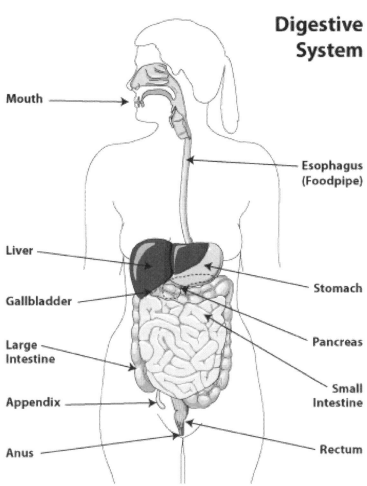

Digestive System

Mouth

Esophagus (Foodpipe)

Liver

Stomach

Gallbladder

Pancreas

Large Intestine

Small Intestine

Appendix

Anus

Rectum

Table Of Symptoms

Here's a list of just some of the health conditions that can and will respond very well to the strategies I will be revealing in this book:

Asthma

Eczema

Urticaria (hives)

Rhinitis (seasonal and perennial)

Catarrh and sinusitis

Gas, flatulence

Abdominal bloating

Arthritis (all types but especially rheumatoid)

Lack of energy and ambition

Inability to think clearly (foggy brain of "woolly" brain)

Behavioural disorders in children

Dizziness

Panic attacks

ADD, ADHD

Autism

Learning disorders

Colitis and Crohn's disease

Eating disorders (anorexia and bulimia)

Diarrhea

Constipation

Haemorrhoids

Headaches

Hypertension

Mastitis or breast pains

Meniere's disease

Migraine

Mouth ulcers

Multiple Sclerosis

Myalgic encephalo-myelitis or Fibromyalgia

Polymyalgia

Pre-menstrual tension

Psoriasis

Recurring Cystitis

Alcoholism

Anxiety

Depression

Violent behavior, smashing up attacks

Frigidity

Hypothyroidism

Impotence

Nephrotic syndrome

Schizophrenia

Depression

Alzheimer's disease

Parkinson's disease

Cardiac arrhythmias (especially tachycardia)

Angina

High moods

Low moods

Variable moods

Hypertension

Overweight

Underweight

Variable weight

Hyperhydrosis (excessive sweating, not related to exercise)

Abnormal fatigue, not helped by rest

Nosebleeds

Diabetes (both types but especially type II)

(With acknowledgements to Theron Randolph, Richard Mackarness, Vicky Rippere and Marshall Mandell)

That's not to say all these conditions are wholly, 100%, caused by "fire in the belly" (though some are). But as I said, the influence of the extreme high level of intestinal inflammation that is present in humans today is such that, once it is corrected, many of the more serious conditions will regress or, quite often, disappear altogether.

Once you understand the character process of inflammation and the "overload" and target organ phenomenon (page 8) you will understand why this is so.

Other Disease Models

I don't want you to misunderstand a list like this or how it works. These are really symptoms and diseases related to a body in overload; that is, stressed outside its comfortable, working physiological and metabolic range.

Not one of the conditions from this list is concretely indicative of a food or chemical allergy, or any other cause of inflammation. So it would be wrong to light on, say, an eating disorder, overweight or depression and say that must be caused by a food allergy or intolerance.

It's really about quantity. The truth is that the *more* items from this list you suffer from, the more likely it is to be an overload of the kind I'm writing about. One or two items would be suggestive; five, six or seven, make it probable. A person with a skin rash and fatigue, with occasional bouts of abdominal bloating and diarrhea, I would say, very likely has "fire in the belly" and would be well advised to check out the possibility, using the methods I give in this book.

It's also about appropriateness. If someone was depressed and lethargic, with no real reason; for example, he or she had a good life, without lack of material goods and has a loving partner or spouse, it's worth checking this out. Many a marriage has been saved by following the route I lay out in this book.

Neither is this meant to exclude other working health models. For example, many practitioners who know their stuff (I mean *really* know their stuff), when confronted with eczema would think of a "hot liver"; a Chinese traditional medicine specialist would think

> Many a marriage has been saved by following the route I lay out in this book.

of too much Yang or deficiencies in the lung and kidney systems; a classically-trained homeopath would certainly think of a sulfur constitution; and a good counselor would ask about stress.

Using a treatment modality from these other models might also produce a good result. That would not make it unlikely that "fire in the belly" was present. Over forty years as a clinician, I can tell you that disease always has multiple causative components, never just one trigger. Food and bowel inflammations are one of the commonest of all contributive factors to a whole host of diseases and mental states.

Maybe it would still be wise to check out the possibility of "Fire In The Belly", at the earliest possible convenience.

Five Cardinal Symptoms

Dr Richard Mackarness, author of the food allergy pioneering book *Not All In The Mind*, gives five key symptoms that point the way to allergic illness and that have special importance. He believes that without one of the following symptoms diagnosis of an inflammatory or intolerance food is unlikely:

1. Over– or underweight or fluctuating weight

2. Persistent fatigue that isn't helped by rest.

3. Occasional swellings around the eyes, hands, abdomen, ankles, etc.

4. Palpitations or speeded heart rate, particularly after meals

5. Excessive sweating, not related to exercise

It needs mentioning that there should be no other explanation for these symptoms.

The following table lists symptoms commonly encountered with allergies and maladaptation syndrome. The list is far from complete.

It is important to say that most of the symptoms could be caused by some other illness, although several – such as sneezing attacks – are

> What really matters is the number of symptoms – the more of these you have, the more likely it is that your illness is allergic in origin.

11

peculiar to allergies. What really matters is the number of symptoms – the more of these you have, the more likely it is that your illness is allergic in origin.

Some are quite obvious; those denoting digestive disturbance would point particularly to a food allergy in the absence of any other pathology. Those affecting the brain show up clearly as mood changes, altered feelings, etc.

What often surprises people are those symptoms of feeling bad first thing in the morning. This is so common most people can't accept that it is even a disorder, never mind an allergy. It's almost considered normal to feel that way! The key is food addiction. By the time a person wakes up in the morning, he or she has often been off food for 12 to 14 hours: that's enough to start up withdrawal symptoms. He or she then has breakfast, which acts like a 'fix' and symptoms start to clear. Certainly these feelings are common, but that's only because masked food allergies are very common.

Another surprise is the 'four – day flu', which isn't really flu at all – it's a food allergy. Dr Arthur Coca, another pioneer of allergy detection and treatment, said, 'You don't catch colds, you eat them'. He had a point: a person eats a food, symptoms are centered on the nose and muscles so he or she experiences headache, runny nose, aches and pains, maybe even a temperature, but a few days later, when the food leaves the bowel, the symptoms disappear. That's too quick for the natural course of a viral disease.

My Own Number One

To me, the number one symptom of an inflammatory food (or any other allergy or overload) is: **Abrupt changes of state from being well to unwell (well one minute, sick a few hours later, then back to well in a day or two).**

The fact that symptoms are there sometimes and not at others make certain types of disease very unlikely to be the cause of sickness: tumors, degenerative disease, genetic disease and infections (just about all the rest) simply do not have the pattern of coming and going over the space of a few hours, or even days.

Ingesting an inflammatory food or inhaling an allergen or sensitized chemical will, however, present in just that way.

There is a plus to this, which I used to explain to my patients, which gave them a lot of comfort. In fact it was a dictum you should learn: **if you can be well one day, you can be well every day!**

By that I mean that if there were good days with few or no symptoms—and that's the common picture, not continuous sickness—then the patient has nothing busted, nothing missing, not a tumor or some crawly parasite. In other words, no reason to not feel continuously well, once the trigger causing symptoms was found and eliminated.

This can be startling too. I cannot count the times I have had a patient come to the office with an x-ray, showing arthritic changes (for example), and telling me at length that this was the "reason" they had unpleasant aching joints.

But then I ask him or her, "Do you ever have pain free days?" If the answer is yes, then how can the joint changes on x-ray be the real reason? In fact I have put patients on a hypoallergenic diet, to settle down the belly fire, and watched the supposed pain of arthritis vanish in 24- 48 hours. How can that be?

The x-ray changes were still there! So clearly the contented certainty that doctors use to fuel their scientific smugness is open to question. They don't even ask elementary logical questions of this sort, and so never come to understand that their "explanations" are often just a bunch of hooey (Oops, went American just for a moment there!)

We Listened To The Patient!

Most of what I learned, I learned by listening and watching. My army of patients taught me almost everything of importance over a period of three decades. There was no formal body of data and very little published in this area. I tried myself to fill in with a few popular paperbacks for the mass market.

At no time did I have the desire to try and persuade my colleagues they were missing something important. The medical profession has a peculiar resistance to change, which seems out of step with the high calling of a physician. This resistance, despite curricular revisions, has led to what has been dubbed "reform without change".[3]

The typical MD, who prefers to believe his textbooks and ignorant peers, does not acknowledge what his eyes and ears tell him. He or she will not listen to patients and so misses the abundance of clues that just talking to a patient would serve to them.

The times I heard a patient say with a sigh, "Every time I drink milk I get a migraine; I told the doctor but he said it was nonsense" and similar expressions of dismissal and dismay are legion.

Because these patients didn't fit into the textbook-defined syndromes or disease patterns, doctors would simply dismiss the patient as a fool, faker or malingerer. They never question their own teachings; only the patient's sanity. Indeed, the aforementioned UK psychiatrist Richard Mackarness wrote his paradigm-bending book entitled *Not All In The Mind*, precisely because of this common attitude towards unhappy patients, that they must be imagining their symptoms and their complaints were therefore all in the mind.

It never seemed to occur to such doctors that it was a measure of their own incompetence that they could not help, rather than an indication of patient trumpery.

They were simply not asking the right questions or doing the right tests!

Shock organs

The trouble was, they were on the wrong model. An absolutely VITAL part of medical grammar was missing from their language altogether and that is the concept of target or shock organs.

A knowledge of this model changes everything a doctor knows (or thinks he or she knows) about health and disease.

The orthodox doctor is used to the idea that one pathogen gives rise to one symptom, or cluster of symptoms (called a syndrome). If you know the pathogen, you know the predicted symptom cluster— "Patient doesn't have that: he/she is therefore a fraud. Ends."

What we pioneers found is that the symptom does not necessarily depend on the pathogen but on the part of the body that breaks down and malfunctions as a result. *The organ most affected will most predict the symptoms that result.*

We speak of a target organ or shock organ. Technically, we can use the term **end-organ failure** or overload.

Thus a milk allergy could cause a rash, if it hits the skin; a wheeze if it hits the lungs; an ache if it hits the joints; or colitis if it hits the gut; and so on. See diagram for examples of target organs and related symptoms.

Probably no recent development in the study of allergy has caused more confusion than the recognition of the multiplicity of symptoms it can produce. No doubt this has hampered progress, since the traditional medical view of patients

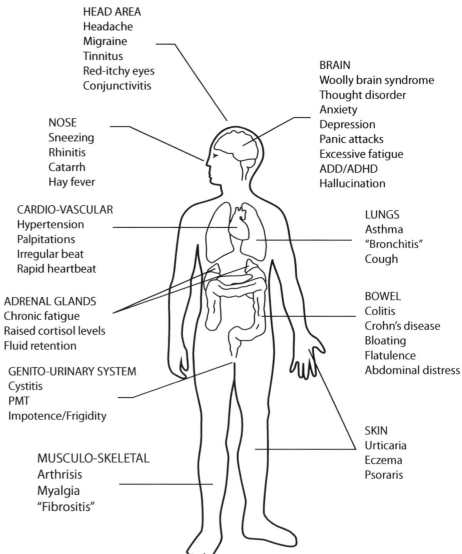

HEAD AREA
Headache
Migraine
Tinnitus
Red-itchy eyes
Conjunctivitis

BRAIN
Woolly brain syndrome
Thought disorder
Anxiety
Depression
Panic attacks
Excessive fatigue
ADD/ADHD
Hallucination

NOSE
Sneezing
Rhinitis
Catarrh
Hay fever

CARDIO-VASCULAR
Hypertension
Palpitations
Irregular beat
Rapid heartbeat

LUNGS
Asthma
"Bronchitis"
Cough

ADRENAL GLANDS
Chronic fatigue
Raised cortisol levels
Fluid retention

BOWEL
Colitis
Crohn's disease
Bloating
Flatulence
Abdominal distress

GENITO-URINARY SYSTEM
Cystitis
PMT
Impotence/Frigidity

MUSCULO-SKELETAL
Arthrisis
Myalgia
"Fibrositis"

SKIN
Urticaria
Eczema
Psoraris

with many and variable symptoms has always been that they were somehow neurotic and 'putting it all on'.

Some doctors like to use the term 'pseudo-food allergy syndrome', which does not help patients at all. One of the sacred texts of this disagreeable nonsense appeared in the Lancet in an article by D. J. Pearson, K. J. N. Rix and S. J. Bentley entitled 'Food Allergy: How Much is in the Mind?' (Lancet i: 1259-61, 1983). Pearson, incidentally, is the man who kept a dossier on me in the early 1980s!

The trouble is, these researchers made no allowance for the fact that their tests might be at fault and assumed, because they got no reaction, that the patient was deluded. Yet their tests were the equivalent of evincing the effect of eating a beef steak by allowing the patient only two capsules of beef.

This is not to say that there are no neurotic individuals whose symptoms might be an attempt to win sympathy from a world they find too hostile; merely those such people are in a small minority.

The Brain As A Target Organ

The number one target or shock organ, which gets hit in almost every case, is the brain and the results of this can be incredibly complex and fascinating.

Many universal symptoms are often a result; fatigue being the outstanding one. The fiery food or pathogen excites the brain, which goes into overdrive and then pretty soon packs up exhausted. Thus revving your grey matter with caffeine all day is a pretty dumb act; it will lead to nervous exhaustion, which then requires more caffeine to get it firing again, and so on, round and round in a vicious cycle.

A popular caffeine drink likes to popularize the slogan "you can sleep after you are dead." Too bad they are not compelled to warn youngsters that this final sleep will come sooner, rather than later, if those who drink it do not observe sensible health measures.

Quite apart from brain stimulation or fatigue, other symptoms can take on an incredible shifting variety of patterns. The brain is the organ which summates our principal sensations and interprets them. Any toxic overload can lead to hallucinations, excitation, mania and hyper activity; the reverse, which often follows quickly, leads downwards, through increasing fatigue, inertia, depression, slowing down and finally coma.

I have seen allergies (food and environmental) lead to heightened sexual feelings, murderous assault, schizophrenic psychosis, woolly thinking, hallucination, hyperactivity, depression, anxiety, learning difficulties, dyslexia and autism spectrum disorder.[4]

But it becomes more complicated than this. Allergies, inflammation and overload conditions can lead to the mechanism of maladaptation, meaning an addiction to toxic substances (more of the full mechanism later).

The main characteristic of addictive phenomenon is that symptoms are relieved by a "dose" of the addictive substance. A heroin user does not shoot up because it makes him or her feel bad; the habit is driven by the fact that he or she feels better, because it relieves the terrible withdrawal symptoms, albeit only temporarily.

> Many universal symptoms are often a result; fatigue being the outstanding one.

So it is with inflammatory foods and allergies of many kinds: eating the food relieves the related symptom, so further adding confusion to the picture. When I hear somebody say "I like a cup of tea; it soothes my nerves", I know straight away that tea is probably making that person tense and anxious. He or she is drinking it to keep that feeling at bay.

Excluding tea from the diet would bring about a recovery—but only after days of unpleasant withdrawal effects. Recovering from food addiction can sometimes be as bad as heroin "cold turkey". I have seen individuals lie on the bed and shake uncontrollably for days, the stink of sweat and fear carried down the corridor, until the foodstuff finally cleared the bowel and blood and the patient felt well again.

So here then is a double whammy: the effects of eating the food and getting overload symptoms, complicated by the effects of not eating the food and getting withdrawal symptoms!

No wonder this took a good deal of work to figure out and we may always be grateful to US pioneers (Sr. and Jr.), Albert Rowe, Arthur Coca, Herbert Rinkel and Ted Randolph (more of them later).

Protean and Bizarre

The truth is that brain overdrive or fatigue states can lead to hundreds of symptoms, if not thousands. Some of these are protean, bizarre, variable and subjective (doctors don't like the word subjective in this context: if only one patient gets it, they react with suspicion that this cannot be a *real* symptom!)

But really, if the patient were to imagine things, is that too not just another symptom? I mean, duh!

Examples of such bizarre and subjective responses I have seen over the years include things like "hot water running down the inside of my skin", "feeling like I am seeing the world down a long, dark tube" and "feeling dirty and wanting to strip my clothes off".

Protean is just an old-fashioned word that means changeable; like the mythic figure of the Greek sea-god Proteus. He would appear in many different forms, such as a man, a beast, a seductive siren, and so on. In this case the patient would visit the doctor one week with headaches; next week it would be diarrhea or colic; the week after, nightmares and hallucinations; a month later excessive fluid retention. So the doctor would inevitably label such patients as hypochondriac and symptoms therefore "all in the mind".

But somatic reactions too can be subjective. I have had many patients whose epilepsy traced to brain excitation from fiery allergy foods. Not too surprising, except that nobody else seemed to recognize it!

But the point is we don't all convulse when we eat our foods. It's a very idiosyncratic response, though I am reminded of the wise words of Professor John Soothill, of Great Ormond Street (we were supposed antagonists but I enjoyed my brief conversations with him); Soothill said "the really amazing thing is not that some patients sometimes react to foods; it's that we don't all react to all of them, every time we eat."

He was making the point that, in our primitive understanding of the day (1983), we ought to be mounting a violent antigen-antibody response to the foreign proteins of every food we eat. But that didn't happen.

What You Don't Eat Is Crucial

Because of the above confusions and seeming contradictions, most doctors have not connected with what is going on inside their patients. If he or she did, then dietary changes would be the first order of business in any medical consultation, even with serious diseases such as heart attack, cirrhosis and cancer.

It's also the basis of my own dictum and revised understanding of nutrition, at least for well-fed developed countries that: **it matters more what you are eating that you shouldn't eat, than what you are not eating that you should** (just in case that came out a bit garbled, let me re-state it: what you should STOP eating has far more impact on your health than what you should START eating.

That's why some diets work well: they, in effect, exclude a troublesome food from the person's diet.

But often the ignorant or unwary doctor, practitioner or nutritionist believes that their choice foods are "doing the person good".

In fact not eating at all (fasting) is also seen to have the same dramatic benefit, for those who take the trouble to work round their ignorance and prejudice and actually figure out what's really going on! So avoidance is definitely the key.

I repeat: what's going on down there in the gut is far more fiery and pathogenic than we ever imagined and what you do NOT eat is of far more concern for your health. "Good foods" are really, simply displacing the bad ones.

There are molds and yeasts (related to Candida) in our diet, too.

I'll come to the latest research on that theme shortly and in detail in chapter 5, The Human Microbiome. It's much more exciting and far-reaching than you could possibly believe.

Let me just fill out the main outline of these discoveries by going on to say that, early in the 1970s and then 1980s, some of us began to see another side to "fire in the belly"; not so much what we were eating but what's living down there in the dark and moist caverns of our gut!

Dysbiosis

It started with Dr Orian Truss and the Candida story back at the end of the 1970s. Some ignorant practitioners and "experts" have never really got beyond this stage. But, trust me, it's much bigger than that.

There are molds and yeasts (related to Candida) in our diet, too. Not just in cheese and mushrooms – unwanted molds. Moreover there are baker's yeast and brewer's yeasts; the former is used in bread and cakes but brewer's yeast is found more widely distributed than merely alcoholic drinks: it's in sauces and foods of all kinds.

Bread is a shocking and surprising avenue of exposure. In 1980 the following fungi were found in flour milled in the UK: *Penicillium, Cladosporium, Aspergillus candidus, Aspergillus flavus, Mucor, Aspergillus terreus, Alternaria, Aspergillus versicolor Absida, Aspergillus fumigatus, Verticullium* and *Paecilomyces* (Food Surveillance Paper, HMSO, no 4, 1980).

Mold contamination of animal feeds can lead to further exposure. Both molds and toxins (along with antibiotics, hormones and sedatives) pass into dairy produce, meat, eggs, bacon and poultry.

As the molds' main port of entry is the mouth, the digestive tract tends to be the most affected. Darkness and moisture within the gut suit these organisms very well. Add to that the fact that our immune systems seem to be already under siege and, not surprisingly, we have a formula for trouble of epidemic proportions. Malabsorption syndrome develops due to intestinal inflammation together with an inability to eliminate cellular waste.

As my friend Dr Nancy Dunne in Dublin was inclined to put it, pseudo-celiac disease with negative alpha-gliadin antibody titres and normal jejunal biopsy but full symptomatology is now as rife as the common cold.

Genetic Food Intolerance

Now it gets more complicated. As the decades rolled by, science progressed. The discovery of the DNA by Watson and Crick was fascinating. An inheritance code? So everyone thought.

But things were supposed to be miraculously revealed to us with the decoding of the full human genome; that is, unraveling the sequence of coded genes in a strand of DNA, which goes to make up a human being, completed in 2003.

The first shock is that we only have 20,000 – 25,000 genes! Aw, c'mon: it's not possible to code a human being in so few bits of information. In fact, 35% of our genes are the same as a daffodil. So we only have 12,000 – 15,000 human genes…

In my opinion, the whole theory of genes coded in DNA is bunk and has today been shown as such. I prefer the model I shared in my book *Virtual Medicine*: that DNA is an energy and information transmitter (it has the characteristics of a fractal arial, perfect for transmitting complex biological messages).

That's not the point here. The other BIG shock was to discover that we have countless tiny variations in this supposed "human genome". So much so, it's true to *say nobody has the human genome; not one human being!*

Instead, we all have little variants called single-nucleotide polymorphism or SNPs for short (which we pronounce "snips"). Translation: a nucleotide is a tiny chunk of DNA, one of eight, including the four basic molecule units, arginine, guanine, cytosine and taurine, which we can abbreviate to AGC and T.

A typical gene might be sequenced TTCGAAGC. But sometimes little switches occur and this set might be altered to, say, TACGAAGC. Not much of a change; not enough to grow two heads! But it could be enough to make the difference in whether you can tolerate beef or not.

So now we realize that a lot of what we once loosely called "allergy" is actually genetic incompatibility with certain foods. They don't suit us. These foods can't be metabolized properly AND WILL PROBABLY CAUSE INFLAMMATION.

If Only It Was So Simple!

But it isn't dear reader. It's even more complicated today. The problem is that what our genes tell our body to do and not do is only a fragment of our living physiology! We are surrounded by a sea of other genes, which outnumber our own, a hundred to one or more. These other genes come from our food and our bowel flora and also have physiological effects on our metabolism.

Incredible but true.

I know in part this because I found myself, without understanding why or how, controlling or even curing so-called genetic diseases. We could switch genes on and off. We learned epigenetics long before Bruce Lipton claimed to have "discovered" it or the word was even coined.

Now we have realized that food genetics is a far bigger and more complicated process than we ever dreamed. These are exciting times! When we swallow our foods, a whole host of gene material is released into our blood.

Our foods and our bowel flora literally become part of our own genetic makeup in ways which is just far beyond anything we imagined 30-40 years ago.

In a landmark study by Chen-Yu Zhang and his colleagues at Nanjing University in China, it was found that the food we eat shows changes the behavior of your genes in ways that are new to science.

In what is the strongest evidence yet that the genetic material in food survives digestion and circulates through the body, fragments of plant RNA have been found swimming in the bloodstreams of people and cows. Immediately, conventional scientists and journalist have gone wandering off in the direction of "discovering" or "inventing" plant foods which they say will change our genes for the better.

But wait a minute, if natural foods we already have can do that, why not use them? I think it shows that they are still missing the point, slightly.

The genetic material in question is microRNA - tiny strands of RNA, is found in almost all cells with a nucleus and travels from cell to cell in the blood. Zhang and his colleagues wondered whether all the miRNA strands in our blood are made by our cells - or whether some comes from our food instead.

So the team drew blood from 31 healthy Chinese men and women, and also from cows. They treated the samples with sodium periodate, an oxidising agent that modifies mammalian miRNA, so that it cannot be sequenced, but leaves the plant versions untouched. As a result Zhang found some 30 known plant miRNAs floating in the blood of the people and cows.

Zhang is unsure how the miRNAs escape unscathed from the caustic soup of digestive fluids and enzymes in the gut. But substantial research suggests that not all genetic matter from food dissolves in the stomach and intestines. Well, we've been telling them about what we called "leaky gut" for years and they were not interested.

But we knew that food material survived digestion and was responsible for setting up inflammation in the intestines. But it is also absorbed and carried via the blood to remote tissues. So, as I have been saying, the "fire in the belly" is really a systemic event that only starts in the belly.

That plant miRNA survives digestion and circulates through the body was surprising enough. But Zhang wanted to know whether plant miRNA remains functional in animal blood.

For example, a particular gene labeled 168a can alter gene expression by binding to strands of messenger RNA and preventing enzymes from translating the strands into a protein. Zhang's team found around 50 genes that 168a might turn up or down, including the gene for LDLRAP1, that removes "bad cholesterol" from the blood.

So, varied from the old already-out-of-date story that our genes create who we are and how we function. It has become increasingly clear we are all a composite of genes, of which food and organisms in the gut are a far greater proportion than our own human-ness! Sorry, Watson and Crick! You're out!

More on this is a later chapter. Just suffice it to say this gene thing is the biggest breakthrough since anesthetics, antibiotics and heart transplants: and far more universal in applicability.

The fire in our bellies has moved to a whole new ball game in complexity.

For example, cosmetics researchers recently suggested that a pill containing a mix of food extracts can influence our genes and boost collagen production in the skin, reducing the appearance of wrinkles (New Scientist, 24 September, p 10).

A whole new science is born in the field of human metagenomics, a study of shifting genetic populations upon and within our bodies. We are truly a composite, with over a hundred times more genes present than just our human measly ration. We are composites! And most of what happens, takes place in the gut, that dark, moist cavern inside of us (which is technically not inside us at all, but equivalent to the hole of a donut, not the donut itself!)

Hippocrates was right, Rinkel et al were brilliant.

My controversial career was exonerated.

A whole new science was born.

Chapter 2 My Part In This Adventure

To be frank, I can boast being a pioneer in this field, if not actually one of the founding fathers. Credit for the latter goes mainly to three outstanding US physicians: Herbert Rinkel MD, Theron Randolph MD and Michael Zeller MD, who did their investigations in the 1930s and 40s.

> You can rely on my experience when I tell you, food inflammatory reactions in the gut can be a disaster!

The culmination of their work was published in an important but almost forgotten book FOOD ALLERGY (Randolp, Rinkel and Zeller, 1951). They found that almost any food could be the originator of an inflammatory process and that these allergy or intolerance reactions were idiosyncratic, meaning different for everyone.

Before that there were a few stray voices, including the two I mentioned in the opening paragraphs of the book. But others worth mentioning are Sir Robert Burton, Arthur Coca MD, Albert H Rowe, MD, and his son Albert Rowe, Jr., MD, Joseph Miller MD, Richard Mackarness MB BS, Doris Rapp MD (still living), Jonathan Brostoff MA, DM, DSc(Med), FRCP, FRCPath, FIBiol (still living) and last but not least, Prof. William Rea MD (still living).

I rate the discovery that everyday foods can wreak havoc and cause serious diseases as an outstanding major medical discovery, almost on a par with anesthetics and antibiotics. It was the key that opened the door to countless recoveries.

Those great investigators, and we who followed close behind, popularizing it as practicing doctors, created a movement that became called clinical ecology. Later we found too many medically untrained hangers-on adopted the title, for spurious credibility, so we later reverted the name to allergy and environmental illness.

I myself drove a grand furrow, writing and broadcasting the good news all over the world. Lots of discoveries and amazement flowed out of my clinic, including bizarre cases, such as a girl made drunk on potato, a boy whose epileptic fits were caused by eating any food from the carrot family (parsley, dill, celery, fennel, etc.) and a woman suffering migraine headaches most days, from licking office envelopes (corn starch gum).

The satisfying corollary to these, and countless other stories, is the same: they made a FULL recovery, once the origin of their condition was found and eliminated from the diet. It reinforced one of my own adages, which is that the person gets to make the true diagnosis that solves the problem! Meaning, I was correct in my diagnosis of the "fire in the belly", because the patient was cured after taking the necessary precautions.

In 1987 I made international medico-legal history, when a UK Crown Court accepted my testimony that food intolerance leading to brain allergic reactions could make a youth murderously violent. By 1990, the European newspapers and

TV were calling me the world's "Number One Allergy Detective" (a term started by Archie Mackay of the Sunday Mail).

So you can rely on my experience when I tell you, **food inflammatory reactions in the gut can be a disaster!**

How Common Is It?

Just about universal. Even an individual with some years or decades clear of the problem can go on to develop new issues or revert to an earlier ill-health status, due to the re-igniting of "fire in the belly". This can arise as a result of a course of antibiotics or even just a simple viral infection (see especially page 60 Polanksy). So nobody is completely safe from this.

I made the point strongly when interviewed by the BBC, on publication of my second book in 1986. I claimed everyone has the problem to a degree; it's just that people don't know it and doctors don't teach it (because they don't know it, either).

Unknown to me, before the interview, Nancy Wise of the BBC World Service had sent a reporter with a roving microphone out onto the street of London, and she started asking people about food reactions. To everyone's astonishment, about 80% of those stopped admitted reacting to food in some way.

Most people didn't even think about allergy or disease at that time (it took me two decades of public education to make everyone more aware of the phenomenon of food allergy and intolerance). The replies the reporter got were things like: "I don't eat celery, it makes my fingers swell," and "Chocolate gives me headaches."

But of course these really are food reactions and pathological states, however trivial. Maybe you know of reactions to food that you or a loved one suffers from?

Food allergies and intolerance are very common. I put it as high as 80% of patients with symptoms. The good news is that this is often a simple entry point to the case: giving up offending foods often produces a dramatic cure, even from such apparently unrelated conditions as irregular heartbeat, lupus and schizophrenia.

That's not to say the entire cause was a food allergy. But reducing body load is the greatest healing paradigm I know. It works every time…

Other Causes Of Fire In The Belly

Food reactions, we pretty soon found out, were only the half of it. All kinds of other agents could set up inflammation, in the bowel and elsewhere in the body.

These include: molds, chemicals, heavy metals, parasites, resistant bacteria, Candida and other yeasts. I'll be discussing each of these in turn and what to do about them but it is vital that you grasp right from the start that there are a great many things assaulting your bowel and, to paraphrase a remark made to me by a former antagonist, Prof. John Soothill of Great Ormond St Hospital (London), "The real surprise is not that these things make some people ill some of the time; it's that they don't make all of us ill, all the time!"

To make it more complicated still, there were many crossovers. People who were easily sensitized to their environment would often have many or most of these problems preying on their health.

Thus I discovered by the early 80s that heavy metal toxicity was probably the number one agent leading to prolonged Candida, mold and yeast sensitivity. In other words, we couldn't easily clean up the Candida without doing a full heavy metal detox.

Sometimes an acute viral illness would precipitate a sensitivity to food which hadn't before been present. This was a clear case of one type of inflammation leading to another, in a cascade or "spreading" effect.

One of the things we all noticed was that exposure to environmental chemicals, as for example in work exposure or being accidentally doused with pesticides from a crop spray plane, would often lead to the onset of food allergies, which then got worse and worse, until a chemical detox was successfully undertaken.

Slow To Change

Of course the medical profession is notoriously slow to adopt any new ideas. It took decades after the pioneering work of Joseph Lister (1827- 1912) before hygiene was fully instigated in the operating theatre; until then surgeons went on operating in their frock coats, often while smoking a cigar!

Anesthetics also took many years to be adopted. In the meantime reactionary dinosaurs went on cutting off limbs (with the patient tied down and screaming till he or she fainted), claiming they had no time for new-fangled notions like pain-free surgery.

Everyone knows the story of Hungarian physician Ignaz Semmelweis (1818- 1865), who had the temerity to suggest that ObGyn doctors should wash their hands, before touching a pregnant woman's privates! It would, he proved, prevent the spread of deadly puerperal sepsis, a condition that was often 100% fatal. But Semmelweis was rejected and scoffed at by colleagues, until the poor man committed suicide. He was one of women's greatest champions.

And the phenomenon of food allergy and intolerance has been similarly fought or ignored. I've had my share of attacks and been dragged before tribunals. In one instance I was found guilty of serious professional misconduct, for associating with journalists in broadcasting my success stories to the world.

In the 1930's Arthur Coca MD observed that the consumption of foods to which a person was sensitive could cause acceleration in the pulse rate. In the course of using the "pulse test" he found that many more medical conditions were caused by food sensitivity than anyone had realized up to that time.

Yet in the second edition of his book, describing the method and detailing his findings, Coca reported that the first edition led to his being criticized by colleagues for trying to expand the field of allergy. [1, p. 68] He also commented upon his ideas meeting "a skepticism so uncompromising that I have not even been invited to demonstrate the new method described herein." [1, p. vii]

Thus, his ideas were not disproven, but simply ignored. But Coca was quite a heavyweight in the allergy field; he was the first editor of the peer reviewed Journal of Immunology. He was not easily discounted.

> I discovered that heavy metal toxicity was probably the number one agent leading to prolonged Candida, mold and yeast sensitivity.

When Herbert Rinkel submitted an article to the Journal of Allergy in 1936 describing the mechanisms and effects of food allergy, it was refused publication.[3, p. 20] In 1951, when Randolph, Rinkel and Zeller published their *Food Allergy* [4] which described a system for detecting food sensitivities in which patients' observable or reported reactions to specific foods could be verified objectively through leukocyte counts of blood samples.

As did Coca, these workers found many more symptoms and illnesses caused by food sensitivities than were conventionally recognized. The typical food reactor is polysymptomatic, "with a long history of many problems, physical and mental," [3, p. 16] the type of person conventional medicine is least successful in dealing with.

At least they were not denied publication and, Randolph especially, published numerous articles in medical journals over a period of four decades.

Nevertheless, clinical ecology remains controversial, and is either unknown or rejected by most allergists, with food sensitivity still being regarded as quite rare. A major problem is that while the immunological basis of allergy as conventionally viewed is well developed theoretically "much of the study of food allergy is empirical practice with no relation to basic science and no knowledge of the pathogenic mechanism involved."

This is nonsense, of course. It is basic science to observe what you observe, correlate it and make deductions. Indeed ALL science is conducted in that fashion. You don't need to know the mechanism to make a scientific observation or speculate on the cause to be valid; think of the present status of the Big Bang theory (entirely unproved speculation).

Physicians are warned against making diagnoses of allergy; one conventional textbook warns that "the allergist should avoid the pitfalls of over-diagnosing allergy," while an editorial in *The Lancet* states that "the diagnosis has been overworked to explain a great array of poorly understood symptoms." [5] The charge that allergy is diagnosed too frequently is based on the conventional view, which is thus used to discourage further examination of alternatives.

What is happening here is that doctors with one view are ignorant and unwilling to consider any other view and believe that, until matters are settled, patients should be left to suffer their fate (good income for the allergists!)

It is basic science to observe what you observe, correlate it and make deductions.

Meantime, in the 1970s and 80s, a handful of doctors like myself rolled up our sleeves and got on with it. Our attitude was "Take as long as you like to make up your minds but until then, we are going to continue serving the patients, by working with them on their food and environmental sensitivities".

I have never regretted doing this and enjoyed the pleasure of tens of thousands of patients, most of whom I was able to help and several of whom have continued to be lifelong friends.

Matters have improved but slightly since then. Really, it has been the impetus given by patients' dissatisfaction and their demands for better solutions than palliative drugs, which has led to the worldwide explosion of interest in food and other allergies.

Meanwhile, orthodox doctors remain ignorant or skeptical. Thus, three researchers in a recent report on the use of sodium cromoglycate (a drug intended to block food allergies) stated they "were surprised to note that symptoms not usually ascribed to allergy, such as lassitude, irritability, rheumatism (aching limbs and joints) and headache were ... produced by the ingestion of foods." [6]

Every one of these symptoms, and many others as well, were ascribed (in at least some cases) to food sensitivity by Rinkel, Randolph, and Zeller in 1951[4] and Albert Rowe MD even earlier. That knowledgeable physicians should find them "surprising" almost thirty years later is eloquent proof of serious resistance to change in the profession.

Interestingly, though, Rinkel's death in 1963 was noted in the Archives of Otolaryngology with a two-page obituary which included his picture and described him as an "internationally known... foremost authority on allergy." [7]

He would have been pleased. I'm sure.

On a personal note, Randolph's description of my first food allergy book (1985) as "the best book of its kind in the world" was a source of immense satisfaction to me.

1.   Coca AF. Familial Nonreaginic Food Allergy, 2nd edit. Chas C. Thomas, Springfield, Ill., 1945

2.   Dickey LD. Clinical Ecology. Chas C. Thomas, Springfield, Ill., 1976

3.   Randolph TG, Moss R. An Alternative Approach to Allergies. Lippincott & Crowell, New York, 1980

4.   Rinkel HJ, Randolph TG, Zeller M. Food Allergy. Chas C. Thomas, Springfield, Ill., 1951

5.   Editorial. Food Allergy and Intolerance. Lancet 2:1344, 1980

6.   Vaz GA, et al. Oral Cromoglycate in Treatment of Adverse Reactions to Foods. Lancet 1:1066-8, 1978

7.   Williams, RI. Obituary, Herbert J. Rinkel, M.D., 1896-1963. Arch of Otolaryngology, 79,1-2,1964

Brain Allergies

I became best known for allergies that affect the brain, largely because of the wealth of strange and interesting cases, which excited media attention. This is one of the less known and probably most significant of all "fire in the belly" reactions, just as Phillipe Pinel said.

In 1987 there was the so-called "Irish Potato Boy". The newspapers loved the story because of the irony of an Irish person being allergic to potato.

Tony Docherty, a Belfast youth, had been charged with attempted murder; he had tried to strangle his step-father. The charge was later mitigated to one of assault. In one of those strange twists of fate, the judge of the Ballymena Crown Court had read an article about my work and sent Tony to my facility, to have him tested.

He was severely allergic to potato, onion, beef and strawberry, as I recall. The potato reaction was outstanding and had Tony sweating and growling; at one point he stood up in front of the nurses and took off his jacket menacingly. I was called to calm him down. All this was filmed by a visiting Channel Four camera team.

The happy outcome was that my evidence that food allergy made Tony potentially violent was accepted by the court. He was not "let off" but was given a conditional discharge: that he sticks to the diet I recommended, otherwise go back to jail!

Thus I made medico-legal history. This was the first time a court of law, anywhere in the world, accepted that food allergy could set fire to the brain!

"I could have saved Marilyn Monroe" was another headline about me in a major British newspaper. I had observed that Marilyn Monroe had classic signs of food allergy. She was already sensitive to fabrics, which I believe was the real reason she liked to be in the nude at home, and not a lascivious nature, as the media liked to portray. But Marilyn also had dreadful hangovers, a classic sign of food allergy, and couldn't get herself started without a couple of Bloody Marys. The vodka would be grain based and addiction to grains and other allergy foods is something that we shall come to in a later section. Heavy withdrawal symptoms would make her feel severely depressed each day, until she got her "fix".

This was the first time a court of law, anywhere in the world, accepted that food allergy could set fire to the brain!

Another large British Sunday paper ran stories of women sexually aroused by reactions to foods. Of course the women didn't know that, till I found out for them! But one woman undergoing a food challenge test, of the kind described on page 83, was overtaken by a strong desire to masturbate. She felt filthy and took herself to the shower. Another woman, it was ice cream I think, grabbed the nearest cooperative male for casual sex and also behaved in an inappropriate and uninhibited manner. A third lady started being suggestive to her husband when I gave her an injection of chicken test extract. I told him, "Forget champagne and oysters; a chicken sandwich will do the job!" We all enjoyed the joke.

It's not that I "set up" these women and others like them, in any way. Their behaviors were quite uncharacteristic. But when tests are carried out using the correct procedure, brain excitation provoked this result. It's much the same as alcohol having a toxic effect in inhibitory pathways. Women who get drunk are notoriously loose and out of control.

A delightful young girl, Josie, appeared with me on Alan Titchmarsh's lunchtime magazine program from BBC Pebble Mill, Birmingham, back in the late 1980s. Josie got drunk, eating potatoes! Really... She slurred her words and staggered, just as if she had imbibed too much. She was intoxicated, without doubt. But not due to drink; due to the toxic effect of this particular food on her brain.

Alan's wit and sensitive questions allowed the whole of Britain to tune in and learn about an otherwise totally unknown phenomenon that puts young women as risk.

The larger issue has been described as "brain allergy" and the consequences can be varied and fascinating. Not just sexual excitation but lethargy and fatigue, low moods, hallucinations, depersonalized states, hypomania and mania, schizoid states, panic attacks, anxiety, violent behavior and a whole host of symptoms that can really be attributed to altered brain function states.

I learned a lot from my great mentor, the late Theron Randolph, who was onto this before the rest of us. He gave me permission to freely use his great concepts in this field and I readily share them with you, feeling that if you truly understand them, you will have a grasp of strange human behavior that is far beyond anything typical doctors and psychiatrists are aware of and something that will give you a powerful insight into the behavior of others.

The Ups and Downs of Addiction

Randolph's basic model is of brain excitation, followed by suppression. This is much like the trajectory of an alcohol drinker: at first he or she is aroused, maybe to the point of excessive behavior. But that arousal state is inevitably followed by a period of extreme drowsiness, even followed by coma, if severe.

And in fact you can follow this sequence with most food allergics, watching them become alternately aroused and later stuporose, just like the effect of alcohol.

In the bigger whole-life picture, you see the whole thing echoed in a longer time frame: a child is hyperactive (ADHD) when young and then in later life suffers from extreme lethargy and depression. When once they couldn't be restrained and kept quiet, as the years go by that same food allergy reaction leads to a difficulty in arousing the person or getting him or her interested in life.

Foods that once led to brain arousal, eventually lead to fatigue and low mood, just as a shot of heroin, which may once have been thrilling and arousing, eventually ceases to work; but if the addict incautiously seeks to keep the thrill going, with higher and higher doses, he or she risks that final coma and death.

Just in case you are wary about this, I am not alone in this brain allergy thing. Doctors William H Philpott and Dwight H. Kalita in their powerful book *Brain Allergies* shared numerous similar and revealing cases:

> Hyperactivity in a child being caused by string beans; violent anger in a woman that was triggered by oranges; sensitivity to wheat in a seventeen year old who had been classed as mentally ill for three years; watermelons leading to depression and irritability in a twelve year old; manic depression being caused by milk in a thirty year old patient. Dr Philpott cites many other cases where people's 'psychological' problems have in fact turned out to be reactions to food, chemicals in the environment, preservatives and additives, anti-caking agents in table salt, and chlorinated water.

You may feel sad and confused that this data is not more widely known. As I have said before, doctors are a peculiar profession, where it is unforgivable to be out of touch or ignore developments that could lessen the suffering of their patients. They should wake up to this.

But the ignorance continues in spades. A patient visiting hospital with any number of strange combinations of symptoms is likely to be told there is nothing wrong and it's "All in the mind". Indeed, that was the cue for the title for a famous 1970s book by the aforementioned Richard Mackarness: *Not All In The Mind* (published in the USA as *Eating Dangerously*).

The trouble is doctors are taught to look only for set combinations of symptoms or a "syndrome". Those are considered "real" diseases and anything else, by inference, is therefore not real and the patient must be faking it. It would never occur to these foolish doctors that if they don't do the correct tests and look for the correct causes and conditions, the patient cannot possibly recover.

It is reprehensibly wrong to imply that the patient is therefore the problem.

Trouble is, doctors have barely a clue how wide off the mark they are and how much of the *real* story of health they are missing. For example, most doctors know about inflammation. But they seem to have little idea just how widespread and damaging it can be, interfering with body function at all levels, especially the brain.

After all, the brain controls almost everything else. So fire in the belly, which jumps to the brain, is capable of causing just about anything, any condition, any syndrome or group of symptoms, as we shall see.

Our Second Brain

The enteric nervous system (ENS) or intrinsic nervous system is an independent network and controls the gastrointestinal system. It is a complete network of neurons, neurotransmitters, and special proteins responsible for communications, "thinking," "remembering," and even "learning". The enteric nervous system is sometimes called the "Second Brain" because the esophagus, stomach, small and large intestines are lined with sheaths of tissue containing neurons that contain and work from the same neurotransmitters that exist in the brain and are influenced by these neurotransmitters.

It's not too fanciful a concept.

The enteric nervous system can operate autonomously, just like a brain. It normally communicates with the central nervous system (CNS) through the parasympathetic and sympathetic (autonomic) nervous systems. However, vertebrate studies show that when the vagus nerve is severed, the enteric nervous system continues to function.

The ENS influences mood and can lead to good and bad emotions. It is the cause of those "butterflies" in the tummy and the physical mediator of what we call a "gut feeling".

32

Control Of Digestion

The "real" brain and nervous system exert a profound influence on all digestive processes, namely motility, ion transport associated with secretion and absorption, and gastrointestinal blood flow. But the ENS too has an enormous array of functions, as reflected in its magnitude and complexity; it contains some 100 million neurons, more than in either the spinal cord or the peripheral nervous system!

The ENS is best seen as the 3rd component of the autonomic nervous system, along with the sympathetic and parasympathetic nervous systems.

We don't want to bog down in the anatomy of this but the ENS has two networks, both of which are embedded in the wall of the digestive tract and extend from esophagus to anus:

The myenteric plexus exerts control primarily over digestive tract motility.

The submucous plexus, as its name implies, is buried in the submucosa and its principal role is in sensing the environment within the lumen, regulating gastrointestinal blood flow and controlling epithelial cell function. In regions where these functions are minimal, such as the esophagus, the submucous plexus is sparse and may actually be missing in sections.

Sensory neurons receive information from sensory receptors in the mucosa and muscle. At least five different sensory receptors have been identified in the mucosa, which respond to mechanical, thermal, osmotic (concentration) gradients and chemical stimuli. Chemoreceptors sensitive to acid, glucose and amino acids have been demonstrated which, in essence, allows "tasting" of bowel contents. Sensory receptors in muscle respond to stretch and tension. Collectively, enteric sensory neurons compile a comprehensive battery of information on gut contents and the state of the gastrointestinal wall.

Motor neurons control gastrointestinal motility and secretion, and possibly absorption. In performing these functions, motor neurons act directly on a large number of effector cells, including smooth muscle, secretory cells and gastrointestinal endocrine cells.

So the ENS regulates all aspects of gut function, from breaking down food, absorbing nutrients, and expelling of waste requires chemical processing, to the mechanical mixing and rhythmic muscle contractions that move everything on down the line.

"The system is way too complicated to have evolved only to make sure things move out of your colon," says Emeran Mayer, professor of physiology, psychiatry and biobehavioral sciences at the David Geffen School of Medicine at the University of California, Los Angeles (U.C.L.A.). For example, scientists were shocked to learn that about 90 percent of the fibers in the primary visceral nerve, the vagus, carry information from the gut to the brain and not the other way around.

[Think Twice: How the Gut's "Second Brain" Influences Mood and Well-Being, Scientific American, Feb 12, 2010]

According to Mayer, psychiatrists are going to have to expand to take into account the second brain in addition to the one atop the shoulders. My my, how times change! It makes old Philipe Pinel seem pretty clever (page 8).

Neurotransmitters

Enteric neurons secrete an intimidating array of over 30 neurotransmitters.

Serotonin is perhaps the best known to the layman: the "happy" compound. It may not be that simple and serotonin is certainly pro-inflammatory but in fact 95 percent of the body's serotonin is found in the bowels.

Because antidepressant medications called selective serotonin reuptake inhibitors (SSRIs) increase serotonin levels, it's a common side effect of these drugs to cause gastro-intestinal symptoms. Irritable bowel syndrome also arises in part from too much serotonin in our guts, and could perhaps be regarded as a "mental illness" of the second brain.

There are some weird findings too: serotonin form the ENS may help prevent osteoporosis. In a new Nature Medicine study published online February 7, a drug that inhibited the release of serotonin from the gut counteracted the bone-deteriorating disease osteoporosis in postmenopausal rodents. It is totally counter-intuitive that the gut would regulate bone mass to the extent that one could use this regulation to cure—at least in rodents—osteoporosis.

But it shows we have a lot to learn about our second brain.

Another major gut neurotransmitter is acetylcholine. In general, neurons that secrete acetylcholine are excitatory, stimulating smooth muscle contraction, increases in intestinal secretions, release of enteric hormones and dilation of blood vessels.

But there's also noradrenaline or norepinephrine as the Americans call it, glutamine, gamma-aminobutyric acid and encephalins, plus endorphins and weird stuff you don't need to know about. It's quite a list!

We now have a new specialty: neurogastroenterology. When all is working well, the proficient orchestration of intestinal motility takes place behind the scenes, at an unconscious (autonomous) level. But when it goes wrong, all hell can break loose, including diarrhea, abdominal pain, vomiting, constipation, irritable bowel and… it seems… emotional misery!

Immune Response

The second brain also mediates a lot of the body's immune response; after all, at least 70 percent of our immune system is aimed at the gut to expel and kill foreign invaders.

This needs little comment here, when it comes to infections. But it's important to be aware that food allergies and gluten sensitivity (celiac disease) are also, basically, immune related. Add to that the fact that auto-immune diseases, in which the body attacks its own tissues, is also a disordered immune response and you'll see why the gut, with its massive accretion of immune tissues (Peyer's patches), is so important to our overall health.

To understand this more, let's now learn about this strange manifestation we call inflammation (which literally means "on fire")...

Chapter 3 What Is Inflammation?

The term inflammation (Latin: *inflammare*, to set on fire) means a process of tissue response in the body, which is part of the usual reaction to disease. It's a hot, fiery and often destructive response my title "Fire In The Belly", means simply **gut inflammation** which is a major cause of human ill-health.

"Calor, rubor, tumor and dolor.

However, it is important to bear in mind that inflammation is Nature's intended response. Mostly it's something that we need (acute inflammation). Inflammation is Nature "fight back" mechanism, designed to deal with a threat or invasion. It's only a problem when it is inappropriate and goes on without resolving (chronic inflammation).

Sunburn and chilblains, or the results of a whitlow alongside the fingernail, are familiar experiences of inflammation, which should help you with recognizing its main characteristics.

As every medical student learns in the first semester, the key signs of inflammation are:

Calor, rubor, tumor and dolor. These are Latin words, meaning heat, redness, swelling and pain (you know doctors never like to use plain English when there are complex Latin or Greek names to use instead!)

These four classical signs were described by Celsus, as long ago as 30 BC or so.

Later, another Roman doctor, Galen, is said to have added a fifth sign: *functio laesa*, which means "loss of function" in Latin.

It's more likely that the English doctor/genius Thomas Sydenham coined this last phrase and it was certainly also familiar to Virchow, originator of the "germ theory of disease" (not Pasteur).

It's worth pointing out that these 5 signs are only indicative of surface inflammation—that which can readily be seen on the skin. When the inflammation affects organs deep within, not all of these 5 signs may be apparent. For example, with pneumonia, there may be *no dolor* (pain), because the lung tissue is not fed with sensory nerve endings.

Only when the pleura are involved is pain on breathing apparent (pleurisy).

How Does It Happen?

The inflammatory response can take place due to viral, bacterial or parasitic infections, allergy, trauma, toxins, adverse medications, burns, radiation, cancer, and a variety of other chronic negative conditions.

The main aspects of the process are usually divided into the cellular response and the chemical response. This is a bit artificial, since the inflammatory chemicals come mainly from cells. But we'll stick with it for now.

At the onset of an infection, a burn, or other injuries, certain cells already present in the tissues kick off the process by releasing so-called "mediators", which are responsible for the clinical signs of inflammation.

Vasodilation and its resulting increased blood flow cause the redness (rubor) and increased heat (calor). Increased permeability of the blood vessels, results in an exudation (leakage) of plasma proteins and fluid into the tissue (edema), which manifests itself as swelling (tumor).

Some of the released mediators, such as bradykinin, increase the sensitivity to pain (dolor). The loss of function (functio laesa) is probably the result of a neurological reflex in response to pain.

The mediator molecules also alter the permeability of blood vessels, to permit the exit of leukocytes, mainly neutrophils, into the tissues. The neutrophils migrate to the scene of the crime, as it were, attracted by signaling chemicals called cytokines.

> The main aspects of the process are usually divided into the cellular response and the chemical response.

Acute Or Chronic

Inflammation is usually classified as acute or chronic. Acute means a swift, recent onset, which clears up rapidly. Chronic means, as its name implies, it continues and won't easily go away.

An inflammatory response requires constant stimulation to be sustained. Inflammatory mediators disappear quickly, being easily degraded in the tissues. Hence, acute inflammation ceases once the stimulus has been removed. Acute inflammations generally heal, with little or no assistance.

Acute inflammations would typically include infections, such as a tooth abscess, cystitis and tonsillitis; or a burn undergoing healing.

If constant disturbance is maintained, inflammatory mediators are being produced all the time. Then chronic inflammation is said to have set in. By its nature, chronic inflammation tends to be destructive to the body.

Chronic inflammation is more familiar as colitis, arthritis, diabetes or lupus. Incidentally, the immune cells responsible for chronic inflammation are not the same as those causing the acute or early response.

Not So Clear Cut

Acute or chronic are just convenience terms. The distinction can be blurred. Some diseases have flare up episodes, which then settle down. But these episodes keep recurring through time, so the disease isn't really being resolved.

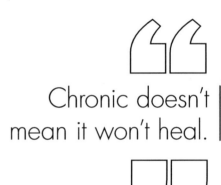

Chronic doesn't mean it won't heal.

Examples would include gout and gall-bladder inflammation; these come and go as flare ups—but won't go away completely unless you remove the cause.

Chronic doesn't mean it won't heal. Any disease can be healed. But the way doctors go about treating chronic disease is based on the belief it can never be fixed and the body is "busted". Therefore it needs some intervention, such as lifelong drugs, as a fix or "patch".

This is nonsense.

All chronic inflammation really means is that the true cause hasn't yet been found. When it is, the patient will recover.

I proved that for myself innumerable times over the years.

Any disease requiring constant medication is, by my terms of reference, not properly diagnosed and being treated ineffectively. The only definition of cure I respect is "no symptoms" (no disease) and "no treatment" (no further medications etc. needed). Chronic medication, just keeping trouble suppressed, solves nothing and is a failure!

Anti-Oxidants Block Inflammation

Most people just don't realize how damaging inflammation can be. If it does not clear up promptly, tissue destruction is almost inevitable. This is because free radicals are flying around while inflammation is taking place.

You may have heard me saying, in other publications, that rapid-fire oxidation (using dreaded free radicals!) is actually how the immune system works. White cells "zap" pathogens with reactive oxygen species, most notably hydrogen peroxide, and then ingest them.

The presence of a plentiful supply of effective antioxidants is essential, to keep the body from injuring itself with these free radicals.

This is even truer when inflammation is calling up lots more free radicals. Thus we would need extra anti-oxidants when inflammation is present. It would be expected that supplementing antioxidant power would actually lessen the signs of inflammation and, in fact, this is exactly the case!

A study published in the journal *Biofactors* in 2004 showed that certain antioxidants effectively reduced inflammation. Of the substances tested, quercitin was by far the best at this, followed by alpha-tocopherol (a species of vitamin E). Beta carotene wasn't much use.

These findings indicate that dietary antioxidants possess significant anti-inflammatory activities, and quercetin is the most potent antioxidant of *those tested*; actually they didn't test a large number of potentially helpful compounds.

[BioFactors, Volume 21, Issue 1-4, pages 113–117, 2004]

Inflammatory Cytokines

Since I went to medical school, it has become abundantly clear that chemical mediators are the main cause of inflammation. In my day, we learned about histamine and bradykinin, which act as potent causes of tissue reddening and swelling. Bradykinin is also a significant cause of pain, when it is released into the tissues.

But since then it has all got much more complicated. Along came a whole host of compounds, known to be part of what is best considered a "cascade" of chemicals, which begin to flow (like a waterfall), where the inflammation is at its hottest.

First came the prostaglandins, PGE-1 (friendly) and PGE-2 (responsible for inflammation). Both of these substances are dependent upon the metabolic pathways for essential fatty acids (EFAs). In simple terms, omega-3s, like DHA and EPA, tend to promote the anti-inflammatory PGE-1 series and omega-6s tend to promote the bad PGE-2 series, which are pro-inflammatory.

That's why fish oil soothes arthritis and donuts make it worse! Fish oils are rich in omega-3s and artificial foods are loaded with disproportionate omega-6s.

But it didn't stop there. We now recognize a host of pro- and anti-inflammatory chemicals called cytokines. Don't get into angst about them. Just get the general idea:

Pro-inflammatory cytokines are the ones that cause inflammation and trouble. The key ones are:

IL-1, IL-6 and TNF-alpha (tumor necrosis factor alpha).

Other pro-inflammatory mediators go on and on and include the IL20 family, IL33 LIF, IFN-gamma, OSM, CNTF, TGF-beta, GM-CSF, IL11, IL12, IL17, IL18, IL8. There are many other chemicals which come into play, attracting inflammatory and immune cells.

The major anti-inflammatory cytokines are IL4, IL10, and IL13.

Other anti-inflammatory mediators include IL16, IFN-alpha, TGF-beta, IL1ra, G-CSF, as well as soluble receptors for TNF or IL6.

These are way beyond the lay person or indeed the average practitioner; I don't know them all, being the province of specialist immunologists. Their interactions are very complex and not fully understood. It is sufficient to understand the concept of "pro-" and "anti-" inflammatory cytokines; being balanced in health but disrupted in common inflammatory diseases.

We'll look more closely at cytokine levels in the section on lab tests for inflammation.

So why is the gut such a potent area for causing inflammations?

Partly, I have hinted, that a large percentage of the immune system is present in the living of the gut. Let's look further into this…

Immunity, or resistance to disease-causing infections, has several aspects.

There is so-called innate immunity: parts of the body which are always on the alert, to keep out invaders. The skin is part of this. Cells called macrophages roam around, munching on anything that comes their way. Tears and saliva contain a substance called lysozyme, which is hostile to organisms. Malic acid secretions in the vagina keep that organ mainly sterile. And so on…

Surprisingly, existing bacteria in the body form what is probably the most powerful barrier to pathogens: harmless bacteria squeeze out the competition, on the same principle that healthy plants help squeeze out weeds and stop them flourishing.

Then there is acquired immunity. That comes from meeting up with pathogens on a previous occasion. This is further split into cellular and humoral immunity.

The cellular element consists of different kinds of white cells, some of which secrete zapper free radicals, some of which secrete antibodies and some of which just gobble up foreign cells (NK or natural killer cells).

The humoral (chemical) element is in the form of familiar antibodies. These are secreted in response to an infection and are designed to specifically knock out a particular protein. Antibodies against streptococcus protein, for example, will incapacitate that strain of bacteria, allowing dead or dying strep to be eaten up by macrophages.

All this sounds rather repetitive, and it is, but I'm parading it here again, to make the point that all this goes on in our intestines, BIG TIME!

> Surprisingly, existing bacteria in the body form what is probably the most powerful barrier to pathogens

Gut Inflammation

The topic that we shall be giving a great deal of attention to in this book is inflammation taking place in the gut. Be aware that over 80% of our immune system lies in the gut.

It starts with the tonsils and adenoids, which are part of this gut protection, before we even swallow.

Lower down there are tonsil-like patches of lymph tissue in the gut wall, called Peyer's patches (named for the seventeenth century Swiss anatomist, Hans Conrad Peyer). These patches are especially abundant in the ileum, the lowest portion of the small intestine.

Peyer's patches contain high concentrations of white blood cells (or lymphocytes). These help protect the body from infection and disease, by detecting antigens such as bacteria and toxins and mobilize white blood cells termed B-cells to produce antibodies.

So the gut is a hotbed of potential inflammation. It's like a mean animal that growls and lashes out at the slightest excuse.

There are several possible triggers and none are rare; food allergy and intolerance is so common as to be virtually the norm. Again, allergy is **an adverse immune response.**

So, are you starting to join up all the dots here?

It amounts to a compelling picture. By far the bulk of immune reactions and inflammatory response are centered in the gut.

There are at least four relevant inflammatory mechanisms, with Peyer's patches right at the thick of it all:
    Food allergy and intolerance
    Leaky gut syndrome
    Dysbiosis
    Heavy metal poisoning
    Improperly digested foods (Indican etc.)

I shall be talking about these at length, later on. Meantime, just understand that food allergy or intolerance is an inappropriate inflammatory response to what should have been safe foods.

Leaky gut is a condition (often started by inflammation) in which the intestine fails to digest food fully to its component molecules and the resulting compounds are absorbed into the blood and set up secondary intolerance and inflammatory responses, often throughout the entire body.

Dysbiosis is the term we use to mean hostile organisms present in the gut which should not be there and which are harmful, by their pathogenic nature. These have arisen because of influences reducing the population of friendly bacteria, such as broad-spectrum antibiotics, too much sugar and other dietary improprieties.

Toxic heavy metals (like mercury) are selectively secreted into the gut and they set up inflammation. This can poison our friendly bacteria, as well as hostile pathogens; impair the function of immune cells; damage the bowel wall and so allow leaky gut; in other words not good news.

Of course there are crossovers too: for example inadequately digested food molecules, not digested well enough to be absorbed across the gut wall, and are acted upon by "unfriendly" bacterial growth in the bowel. When this happens, derivative toxic chemicals, known collectively as "Indicans," are formed. Most of these compounds can be excreted in the feces. However, since they are toxic, they cause a number of problems, not the least of which is inflammation of the bowel itself.

This is a big part of "Fire In The Belly", as we shall see.

Toxic heavy metals (like mercury) are selectively secreted into the gut and they set up inflammation.

"Leaky Gut" Syndrome

Around the mid-80s, we began to recognize the enormous importance of the so-called "leaky gut", an abnormally permeable gut wall, which allowed substances such as toxins, microbes, undigested food, waste, or larger than normal macromolecules to leak through.

The defined space of the bowel (or lumen) contains a considerable immunological and toxic burden, including potentially allergenic food residues, waste toxins, food toxins (both natural toxins and artificially added man-made chemicals), bacteria, parasites and free radicals released by many processes taking place.

It is important to realize that the contents of the bowel are outside the body. If you imagine a piece of string entering at the mouth and emerging from the anus, you will readily see this is true.

It's an area of major interaction with our environment. Although the gut is only 20 feet long, it has a surface area of 3,000 square feet; the equivalent of about two tennis courts. That makes the gut a larger surface area than the skin!

Yet it is lined with only one layer of cells. That means it is pretty vulnerable.

Originally, the idea was that the leaking was caused by increased permeability of the gut wall resulting from toxins, poor diet, parasites, infection, or medications. It was a "wear and tear" effect. To a degree, that remains true.

Then recently, the phenomenon of bacterial biofilm has emerged (page 46). Mostly, this has proved a health danger. But it does appear that there is a "friendly" biofilm, created by our healthy gut flora. It may even be protective and it seems as if, when the biofilm layer is thinned, leaky gut ensues. So the biofilm has a kind of "sealant" effect.

That would explain why dysbiosis might lead to the phenomenon of leaking.

But it's not that simple, it has emerged. Far from being a long-term wear and tear effect, from dietary abuse, infections and poor lifestyle, the leakage is controlled by our new "organ", the enteric nervous system (ENS).

The junctions between the lining cells of the gut wall have been christened "tight junctions". They don't leak much, unless told to! But there is a special signaling system, dependent on a chemical messenger or hormone called zonulin, which is triggered rapidly by firings of the ENS. As zonulin is secreted, the once "tight" junctions open up and leakage is inevitable.

[Wang, W; Uzzau, S; Goldblum, SE; Fasano, A (2000). "Human zonulin, a potential modulator of intestinal tight junctions". Journal of Cell Science 113 (24): 4435–40]

This puts a different face on the hypothesis. For one thing, it's not a long-term damage phenomenon, but an almost instant response which takes place in minutes, not months or years.

At last there is a good physiological model for what we pioneer doctors saw so clearly in the 1970s and 80s: that, after a meal, foodstuffs and immune complexes appeared in the blood and all over the body.

Food as recognizable food gets into the bloodstream and remains identifiable by its immunological source. In other words, "wheat-ness" or "pork-ness" of the food survives. This is then capable of setting up and allergic reaction, to wheat or pork, or whatever culprit is to blame. Even this wouldn't be a problem, if the larger food molecules would only stay put: in the lumen of the bowel.

But they don't.

As a result of increased permeability, the larger immunologically-active molecules escape into the blood, setting up immune complexes (type-IV hypersensitivity, as it's called), and wreaking havoc. The complexes are deposited widely in the tissues, resulting in a systemic inflammatory process, which can affect all parts of the body, including the gut itself. This in turn leads to further loss of integrity of the gut wall and further leakage. Thus food allergy can become a cause of the problem, as well as the result, and a kind of vicious circle is entered.

The model, now better understood, has become a very full one. Yes, a lot of what we encountered was not a true food "allergy", although we fought for the right to call it that. But it certainly was an immune response and there were physical factors entrained in the onset-of-disease process. I'm excited to be presenting this fuller model to the public and explain how crucial it is to all aspects of diet and lifestyle.

Liver Burden

The liver tries to handle these extra-large molecules and remove absorbed toxins, which should have remained behind in the bowel. When this happens the liver is also overloaded, leading to compromise of the cytochrome p-450 detox system (one of the main detox pathways), with resultant escape of toxins, production of excess free radicals and loss of nutritional essentials, such as glutathione and other sulphur-containing amino acids. The liver has to dispose of toxins somewhere and usually this ends up in the bile (most mercury, for example, is excreted into the bile). "Toxic bile" in turn will injure the gut mucosa, trigger leaky gut, and a second vicious circle is in progress. Toxic bile is also known to lead to chronic pancreatitis and possible pancreatic cancer.

[Braganza, J.M., Pancreatic disease: a casualty of hepatic "detoxification"? Lancet, 1983. ii: p. 1000-1002]

But it is worse. For every toxic molecule excreted in the bile, the liver has given up one molecule of precious glutathione, to create a conjugate. That is what is supposed to happen. But when the conjugate enters the bowel and encounters more toxic bile with active free radicals, these attack the conjugate and release the toxin once more. The glutathione molecule is wasted and the toxin is back on the loose.

You will see at once why a diet rich in antioxidants is really essential in combating the chemical plague of our world. We cannot go on squandering our biological reserve in this way, without facing increased risk of cancer and, of course, accelerating the ageing process.

Verifying leaky gut syndrome

A neat and useful model, as I said. But is it valid? A test has been developed to establish whether or not the gut is releasing larger molecules than are biologically acceptable. It concerns absorption of two complex sugars, mannitol and lactulose.

Mannitol is a relatively small molecule and should be absorbed; lactulose is larger and should not be absorbed significantly. The patient fasts and both sugars are administered simultaneously. The information which can be gained is interesting:

- If the absorption of mannitol is low, suspect malabsorption.

- If the absorption of lactulose is high, suspect leaky gut.

- If both are normal, this suggests healthy gut performance.

In fact what is normally measured is the mannitol/lactulose ratio. A recent study published in the Lancet found that the lactulose-mannitol ratio was an accurate predictor of relapse when measured in patients with Crohn's disease who were clinically in remission

[Wyatt, J., et al., Intestinal permeability and the prediction of relapse in Crohn's disease. Lancet, 1993. 341(8858): p. 1437-9]

Biofilms A Second View

Biofilms (bacterial slime and plaque) are widely regarded as a bad thing. They block the access of immune cells and antibiotics to the bacteria which wield them. Biofilm is a sticky mucus substance (an exopolysaccharide, to be technical). In a sense, they are bacterial defence mechanisms. We associate them with dangerous pathogens, like *Pseudammonas* infection.

One of their dangers lies with a clever bacterial enhancement mechanism called "quorum sensing". When bacteria get together in sufficient quantities, they talk each other into doing battle, like a war dance; when they get to a certain frenzy together, they unleash their malice and toxins and start to attack our tissues.

But here again, in yet another thought revolution, we have to face that there is a totally different take on biofilms in the gut. They consist of colonies of good, friendly bacteria, sometimes single species, sometime multiple. These are a good thing and very protective of the gut wall. Evidence shows that when the biofilms are damaged (as with antibiotic therapies), gut inflammation increases. Moreover the gut is more inclined to "leak" (see page 115), once the protective biofilm layer is reduced.

So biofilms actually hold in check that deadly fire in the belly.

Nothing shows the importance of this more clearly than the fact that our own bodies help and support the process of biofilm formation! Our mucus membranes produce helpful antibodies called IgA molecules, secreted by Peyer's patches.

Remarkably, our gut flora have IgA receptors (how is that for evolutionary symbiosis?), which stimulate the secretion of mucin for the biofilm. So it really is true—we help them, they help us.

You can be sure, then, that the healthy body is very adept at recognizing friend from foe and being able to work with the good guys, to shut out the bad guys.

It goes wrong in a number of ways. The most obvious is the use of antibiotics. This clumsy intervention, although lifesaving on occasions, can't help but wipe out good microbes, along with the pathogens. With the balance gone, it's easy for pathogens to take the upper hand.

Being infected by different microbiota is another mechanism. That can be as simple as being intimate with a new lover. Their balance might not suit you so well, or their balance is lopsided and tends to drive your own balance into a distorted pattern.

Thirdly—and by no means the least—our typically bad diet, overloaded with synthetic substances, sugars, other carbs, and depleted of real nutrients is a path to disaster. Add to that the fact that our immune systems seem to be already under siege from xenobiotic chemicals and, not surprisingly, we have a formula for trouble of epidemic proportions, in which the balance of bowel flora cannot help but turn bad.

Darkness and moisture within the gut suit certain mold organisms very well. Malabsorption syndrome develops due to intestinal inflammation together with an inability to eliminate cellular waste, due to loss of helpful symbiotes. As my friend Dr. Nancy Dunne in Dublin was inclined to put it, "Pseudoceliac disease with negative alpha-gliadin antibody titres and normal jejunal biopsy but full symptomatology is now as rife as the common cold"!

A New Role For The Appendix

Now I am going to really shock and amuse you. Remember all that stuff you learned at school, about the useless "vestigial" appendix? We didn't need it any more, they said, it was just an evolutionary hang over. Rabbits had a big one, because they ate their own droppings for food (coprophagia) and this "re-cycled" food was shunted sideways into the appendix for a final digestive fermentation; but humans didn't need ours any longer.

Well, it's just more "science" hooey, which means ignorance and stupidity, instead of fact.

Here is what the appendix is really for: it contains surplus biofilm, from which to recharge our intestines from time to time, with good healthy biofilm.

- The appendix is more than a vestigial organ.

- Evidence indicates it acts as a "safe house" reservoir of healthy bacteria held within biofilms, then used to re-populate the rest of the intestines after stress

- It may be most useful in areas of high enteric pathogen exposure and dysfunctional in "clean" environments, thus explaining the much higher rate of appendicitis in industrialized countries

[The Human Appendix, Journal Of Theoretical Biology 249 (2007) 826 – 831]

You may recognize this is yet another appearance of the "hygiene hypothesis", in which exposure to pathogens, providing we win, is healthier than sterile surroundings.

If you have kids, make sure to tell them that what the biology teacher says about the appendix is bunk!

Auto-Immune Response

There is a further, vicious inflammatory response that causes a lot of illness and suffering. It's called "auto-immunity", a clumsy way of saying that the body attacks itself.

The classic immune response, as you know, is to create antibodies to invasive pathogens. That's how we keep them at bay. Without an effective immune response, we probably wouldn't last more than a day. When the immune system finally fails (full-blown AIDS), we inevitably die and quite quickly too.

But sometimes the body fails to distinguish between the bad guys and the good guys. Allergies, in a sense, are just caused by the immune system generating antibodies to inappropriate substances, like plant particles on the breeze, foods and drink. These are supposedly non-threatening agents.

However, it can be much worse than that. When the process goes really haywire, the immune system can end up attacking our own bodily tissues. We call this "auto-immune disease". It's becoming an epidemic, due to our lousy lifestyles and a toxic environment.

However, in a few types of autoimmune disease (such as rheumatic fever), a virus or infection with bacteria, triggers an immune response and the antibodies or T-cells attack normal cells because some part of their structure resembles a part of the infecting microorganism.

Autoimmune disorders fall into two general types: those that damage many organs (systemic autoimmune diseases) and those where only a single organ or tissue is directly damaged by the autoimmune process (localized). However, the distinctions become blurred as the effect of localized autoimmune disorders frequently extends beyond the targeted tissues, indirectly affecting other body organs and systems.

In some cases, the antibodies may not be directed at a specific tissue or organ; for example, antiphospholipid antibodies can react with substances (phospholipids) that are the normal constituents of platelets and the outermost layer of our cells (cell membranes), which can lead to the formation of blood clots within the blood vessels (thrombosis).

Symptoms of autoimmune disorders vary by the particular disorder but many include fatigue, dizziness, and low grade fever. Symptoms can also vary in severity over time.

The Diseases

The auto-immune process gives rise to a great many diseases; for example, if the body attacks its own joints, we get a certain kind of arthritis called rheumatoid arthritis (this is not the same as the "wear-and-tear" arthritis, which we call osteo-arthritis); when it attacks the thyroid, we get Hashimoto's disease; when it attacks the pancreas, diabetes is the result.

Some of the more common autoimmune disorders include rheumatoid arthritis, systemic lupus erythematosus (lupus), and vasculitis, among others. Additional diseases that are believed to be due to autoimmunity include glomerulonephritis, Addison's disease, mixed connective tissue disease, polymyositis, Sjögren's syndrome, progressive systemic sclerosis, Goodpasture's syndrome (lung and kidneys), some cases of infertility and deadly Multiple sclerosis (MS).

There are other conditions not generally accepted as auto-immune in nature but which one could suspect have that sort of basis; for example, Alzheimer's disease which, in any case, is definitely an inflammatory disease.

Autoimmune Lab Tests

Autoimmune disease if often subtle and not obvious. It may be missed for years, if the physicians look only at organ symptoms. A patient may present with chronic, progressive arthritic symptoms, fever, fatigue, muscle weakness, and/or a rash that cannot readily be explained.

Autoantibody tests may be ordered when an autoimmune disease is suspected.

One test initially ordered is the Antinuclear antibody (ANA) test, a marker of the autoimmune process that is positive with a variety of autoimmune diseases. It may be positive in systemic lupus erythematosus, Sjögren's syndrome, rheumatoid arthritis, autoimmune hepatitis, primary biliary cirrhosis, alcohol-related liver disease, and hepatitis B.

This test is frequently followed up with other specific autoantibody tests, such as anti-Double Strand DNA (anti-dsDNA), anti-Sjögren's Syndrome A (anti-SS-A), anti-Sjögren's Syndrome B (anti-SS-B), Anti-Ribonucleic Protein (anti-RNP) and rheumatoid factor or anti-cyclic citrullinated peptide (anti-CCP) antibodies, which are typically present in rheumatoid arthritis.

Once again, I stress that these are not a concern for the layman. Even the average doctor would not understand half these tests; nor would he or she need to!

In addition, other tests associated with arthritis and inflammation, such as a rheumatoid factor (RF), an erythrocyte sedimentation rate (ESR), a C-Reactive Protein (CRP), and/or complement levels (C3, C4), may also be performed.

During an acute illness, like a severe bacterial infection, levels of CRP quickly shoot from less than 10 mg/L to 1,000 mg/L or more. But in the heart, differences between normal and elevated is so small that it must be measured by a specially designed assay called a high-sensitivity CRP test.

Inflammation experts determined that having a CRP reading of 3.0 mg/L or higher can triple your risk of heart disease. The danger seems even greater in women than in men. By contrast, folks with extremely low levels of CRP, less than 0.5 mg/L, rarely have heart attacks. So there is "Fire In The Heart" too! In fact, it's the major cause of killer heart attacks, NOT clogged plumbing, as the phony cardiac surgeons like to tell you.

See page 40 for more on lab tests for all kinds of inflammatory diseases.

Chapter 4 The Body On Fire

Senility Is Inflammation

Be in no doubt about this. I've been telling you for years. Inflammation is the core of aging. You have to quench that fire to age well.

Senility and dementia also stem directly from inflammation. Those who show signs of inflammation move earlier and quicker into cognitive dysfunction.

It was always thought that in aging our immune systems deteriorate. That's not strictly true. It changes in character. Those who stay fit in mind and body till extreme age have a vibrant immune system. But it is different from that of early life.

> **"Senility and dementia also stem directly from inflammation.**

With age, immune cells called T-cells become more like natural killer (NK) cells, which typically target tumor cells and virus-infected cells. Now a new study that showed people who were most physically and cognitively resilient had a dominant pattern of stimulatory NK receptors on the T-cell surface, and that these unusual T-cells can be activated directly through these NK receptors independently of the conventional ones.

The functionally resilient elders also show less inflammation and signs of a positive functioning immune system.

Conversely, those who aged badly had a dominant pattern of inhibitory NK receptors on their T-cells, and a cytokine profile indicating a pro-inflammatory environment.

Inhibitory NK cells, if you don't get it, means more susceptibility to disease, especially cancer.

All this was demonstrated neatly by a recent study (Oct 2011) from the University of Pittsburg. The findings were published in the Public Library of Science (PLoS).

The researchers concluded that there is remodeling or adaptation of the immune system as we age that can be either protective or detrimental. It's a kind of immunological fingerprint that can identify individuals who are more likely to stay physically and cognitively well.[1]

These findings are supported by other studies, suggesting that people who take anti-inflammatories, such as ibuprofen are less likely to get Alzheimer's, in fact 50% less likely!

It all adds up. Growing old and doddery is inflammation, not wear and tear, genes, telomeres and any of that other stuff. It's fire inside.

Better get those antioxidants down fast, plenty of omega-3s (brilliant against inflammation). And cut the sugar: that's highly inflammatory.

1. Abbe N. Vallejo, David L. Hamel, Robert G. Mueller, Diane G. Ives, Joshua J. Michel, Robert M. Boudreau, Anne B. Newman. NK-Like T Cells and Plasma Cytokines, but Not Anti-Viral Serology, Define Immune Fingerprints of Resilience and Mild Disability in Exceptional Aging. PLoS ONE, 2011; 6 (10): e26558 DOI: 10.1371/journal.pone.0026558

2. http://www.nia.nih.gov/NewsAndEvents/PressReleases/PR1970310AntiInflammatoryDrugs.htm

Suppressing Inflammation

There is a lot to be gained from suppressing inflammation, especially when it affects the brain. I saw some astonishing recoveries in the 1980s and 90s, removing inflammatory foods from the diets of kids with autism. I was one of the leading pioneers, worldwide, in treating autism holistically.

One of the most remarkable stories was that of a young boy I will call Martin (he was from Martinstown, Ireland). He was brought to see me at my facility in Manchester, by his caring and suffering parents. And I do mean suffering—when we joke about needing to nail down the furniture, in this case it was literally true! Martin, age five years, was capable of mustering enough strength to tear a wooden door from its hinges.1

Martin had been quite normal, till his first measles vaccine, after which he suddenly went downhill and deteriorated into a condition known as "disintegrative psychosis". These days we prefer to avoid such pejorative terms. The pleasing part of the story was that, after I identified his food allergens, he made a rapid recovery.

Almost as a direct result of the Martin's parent's experience, I was interviewed on the Gay Byrne Show in Dublin. Gay was a huge media influence at that time, and his word was enough to sway the actions and beliefs of millions.

The response to the discussion on air of food allergies and autism (this is where I first spoke to the media about the tricky question of measles vaccine appearing to be a frequent cause of autism), was that I had a landslide of enquiries. After some consideration, I opened for business in Dublin and spent some of the happiest times of my life in that roaring city!

Case after case of children who recovered well taught me that a wide variety of attention deficit and behavioral disorders were mainly caused by brain inflammation, due to the inflammatory process. It was a cauldron of learning and I saw many remarkable things. Like, for example, young Eamonn. He would write his name backwards (as in a mirror image) after eating wheat or apples. In theory this was a brain disorder but, in trying to imagine the incredible complexity of neurological function needed to write in mirror image fashion, I was impressed! How strange those two foods should cause this weird dysfunction.

By this stage of my career, I knew that reducing inflammation had pronounced positive effects for these cases and simply removing food pathogens was a simple way to accomplish this. It is still the first thing to try. That's why I give the topic such prominence, later in this book.

But now there is another factor in the puzzle, which I learned of long after the Martin adventure. It concerns the so-called "hygiene hypothesis". Doctors and scientists in many countries around the world laugh at developed countries, especially Americans, for their obsession with cleanliness and hygiene. It is their considered view that necessary and continued exposure to pathogens is needed, to keep our immune systems in fully functional order.

Quite simply: no pathogens, means nothing for the immune system to do, so it turns on the body and attacks that instead. The result is the epidemic of auto-immune diseases that we are seeing today.

I have spent time as a doctor in many countries overseas and fully concur with this hypothesis, even though it is unproven.

As with any scientific theory, the way to proceed is to form your hypothesis and then test it. If the hygiene hypothesis is correct, then challenging the body with pathogenic organisms ought to produce detectable benefit in inflammatory disorders, including those which affect the brain and nervous system.

Enter parasitic worms!

The Iowa Studies

In 1982 a team from the University of Iowa began strange new research into the cause of two potentially painful and debilitating inflammatory bowel diseases - Crohn's and ulcerative colitis.

Inflammatory Bowel Disease (IBD) causes many symptoms such as diarrhea, bleeding, abdominal pain, cramps, urgency and loss of energy. These are not nice diseases. They are chronic, relapsing conditions that usually last a lifetime and often seriously impair the patient's quality of life.

Researchers Dr. Joel V. Weinstock, Dr. Robert W. Summers, and Dr. David E. Elliott used tiny parasitic pig whipworms called *Trichuris suis* to dampen the immune system of patients and this benefitted their bowel disease greatly. The fire in the belly was doused!

Initial research on mice showed that the helminth treatment would work. This was followed by a trial involving seven patients, four with Crohn's disease and three with colitis, mainly to confirm the safety of the procedure.

The results were very encouraging. The patients did extremely well and several remained in complete remission for more than two years.

No pathogens, means nothing for the immune system to do, so it turns on the body and attacks that instead.

In a larger trial in 2005, nearly 80 percent of 29 patients suffering from Crohn's disease reported significant alleviation of their symptoms after 24 weeks of treatment.

[R.W. Summers et al., "Trichuris suis therapy in Crohn's disease," Gut, 54:87-90, 2005]

In fact the only real problem was that the whipworm doesn't last long. The body throws them out after a couple of weeks. So constant dosing is required. But that is a small price to pay, for freedom from these debilitating disorders.

The science behind all this is easy: up until the middle of the 20th century, many people lived and worked in a rural environment. They were constantly exposed to farm pathogens, including the pig whipworm, Trichuris. Inflammatory bowel disease was virtually unknown in this population.

The same is still true today in most parts of the world, where billions of people still carry parasitic worms and in those areas - Central and South America, Africa and a large part of Asia - inflammatory bowel disease is almost unheard of.

But then in developed countries, starting in the '30s and '40s, many people left the farms and moved into urban areas, lived in a relatively cleaner environment, and led a nearly sterile lifestyle.

As a result there was an explosion of IBD. The incidence of inflammatory bowel disease has an inverse relationship with the elimination of worms from our environment.

[FASEB J. 2000 Sep;14(12):1848-55. Does the failure to acquire helminthic parasites predispose to Crohn's disease?]

Since the trials of Weinstock's team, this novel protocol has acquired definite scientific credibility, worldwide. The hypothesis is sound, the treatment consistent with the theory and the results are unarguable.

Other workers have published too; for example:

T G Moreels, R J Nieuwendijk, J G De Man, B Y De Winter, A G Herman, E A Van Marck, P A Pelckmans
Concurrent infection with Schistosoma mansoni attenuates inflammation induced changes in colonic morphology, cytokine levels, and smooth muscle contractility of trinitrobenzene sulphonic acid induced colitis in rats Gut 2004;53:99-107 doi:10.1136/gut.53.1.99

I don't think it's necessary to go back to the hygiene standards of the 19th century. But this is a good moment to make the point that soap and water—and especially Chlorox, Dettol and other antiseptics—are not needed. Children should be allowed to play in dirt and not have to wash their hands at every turn.

Hell, when I was a kid in the country we wiped the cow shit from our hands and then held our sandwiches while we ate them, with brown stains on the bread! It didn't seem to do us any harm.

Now, let's go back to autism...

Lawrence's Story

No question the patient, Lawrence Johnson, was in a bad way. By his teenage years, he had veered into the dangerous realm of self abuse. He smashed his head against the wall dozens of times a day. He bit himself until he bled. He gouged at his eyes and tore at his face. A normal school experience was virtually impossible. He couldn't walk a single block from the family's Brooklyn brownstone without kicking and screaming when a traffic light changed at the wrong moment or streets were crossed in an unacceptable order.

Over the years, the Johnsons tried several treatments to curb Lawrence's violent and disruptive outbreaks, including every pharmaceutical that could potentially treat his problems—antiseizure medications, serotonin-reuptake inhibitors, atypical antipsychotics, lithium, and others in various combinations.

At best these heavy medications offered momentary reprieves from what the Johnsons called Lawrence's "freak outs." But any improvements in the boy's behavior were usually short-lived.

[http://the-scientist.com/2011/02/01/opening-a-can-of-worms/ accessed 1/22/2012 2.38 pm PST]

By 2005 the Johnson family was at its breaking point. Something had to be done, or Lawrence would need to be in managed care.

The father trawled PubMed and Medline sites for scientific studies that may help his son's condition. What he found was data that pointed to a link between some autism symptoms and inflated levels of proinflammatory cytokines, an apparent result of the immune system attacking glial cells in patients' brains.

[D.L. Vargas et al., "Neuroglial activation and neuroinflammation in the brain of patients with autism," Annal Neurol, 57:67-81, 2005]

This striking paper is suggesting, in effect, that even autism is a kind of autoimmune disease.

Eventually, Stewart Johnson stumbled across the work of the Iowa group on helminth therapy and how it reduced inflammation, especially the auto-immune type. It was reasonable to hope this might calm his son's outrageous behavior.

Enlisting the help of Lawrence's doctor, Eric Hollander, then the head of Mount Sinai Medical Center's Seaver Autism Center in New York City. Hollander was impressed with Stewart's research and agreed to help him obtain sterile, treatment-grade T. suis eggs that were being grown and tested in Europe by the German company called OvaMed.

It's relatively safe. T. suis has evolved to infect the guts of pigs, and could only colonize humans in a very limited fashion. Like most internal parasites, T. suis cannot complete its entire life cycle in only one host, and in the environment the ova require a 3- to 6-week incubation in moist soil to mature, making inadvertent spread of the parasites to the rest of the family unlikely.

They had Lawrence drink a solution containing 1,000 of the roundworm eggs every two weeks for 5 months beginning in early 2006. The results were very disappointing, to say the least. Lawrence's aggressive and agitated behaviors abated for just four days during the entire 20-week treatment period.

But OvaMed's president Detlev Goj suggested the dose was too small and recommended Lawrence receives 2,500 eggs every two weeks for a period and see what happened.

This time, the results were astounding. Within 10 weeks of the higher-dose treatment, the autistic boy stopped smashing his head against walls. He stopped gouging at his eyes. The paralysis and frustration that held him and his family prisoners in their own home lifted. The freak outs, ceased.

Well, it's a heart warming story. But don't forget: diet, detox and lifestyle modifications come first. These reduce inflammation markedly and often is enough to completely switch off aggressive and disruptive behavior, as in young Martin's case early in this chapter.

To follow Lawrence Johnson's story further, go to this special website: www.autismtso.com

Multiple Sclerosis

Another troubling condition I got to see a great deal of over my clinical years was multiple sclerosis. MS (or disseminated sclerosis or encephalomyelitis disseminata) is an inflammatory disease in which the fatty myelin sheaths around the axons of the brain and spinal cord are damaged, leading to demyelination and scarring as well as a broad spectrum of signs and symptoms

This affects adults more than children. It's a condition that comes on typically at the teens and beyond years. It is more common in women. The prevalence ranges between 2 and 150 per 100,000.

MS was first described in 1868 by Jean-Martin Charcot and I pointed out in my writings over two decades ago that its recognition shortly followed on the introduction of mercury amalgam fillings in Paris. This may be significant.

MS too is clearly an autoimmune-type condition. Environmental risk factors are confusing but have been supposed to include stress, smoking, vaccinations and chemical pollutants. One striking observation is that MS only appears in temperate zones; the further from the equator, the higher the incidence rises.

MS too is clearly an autoimmune-type condition.

Decreased sunlight exposure has been linked with a higher risk of MS, which would fit with lowered sunshine levels far from the equator. Vitamin D may be a protective factor.

Several other possible risk factors, such as diet and hormone intake, have been investigated; however, evidence on their relation with the disease is said to be "sparse and unpersuasive".

[^ a b Rosati G (April 2001). "The prevalence of multiple sclerosis in the world: an update". Neurol. Sci. 22 (2): 117–39. doi:10.1007/s100720170011. PMID 11603614]

I have got so many MS patients back on their feet, using my own protocols, which I am of the opinion that if they investigated diet factors properly, this "unpersuasive" perception would be very different.

An interesting question, in view of the obvious inflammatory nature of MS, is: would helminth therapy help this condition too?

To answer this, John Fleming, a University of Wisconsin neurologist, set out to study 18 patients with MS. Owing to red tape and bureaucracy, it took him many years, from 2004 to 2010 before the

FDA finally gave him clearance Fleming was, in fact, the first researcher to start the application process, and it is to his credit that this made it possible to get the autism trial started.

Meantime, another study was published in Argentina, in which 12 MS patients with naturally occurring helminth infections who were followed for four and a half years showed significantly less neurological damage when compared to 12 MS patients without infections

[J. Correale, M. Farez, "Association between parasite infection and immune responses in multiple sclerosis," Ann Neurol, 61:97-108, 2007]

Food Allergies

If it works in settling down the overzealous immune system, might helminth therapy possibly stifle severe food allergy reactions? Harvard pathologist Marie-Hélène Jouvin, thinks so. She has received permission from the FDA to try TSO for food allergies—and possibly other conditions.

"From what we know from epidemiological studies with helminth infections and from animal studies and from the clinical studies done by Joel Weinstock," she says, "it is clear that there is a good chance that TSO could fine tune or modulate inflammation/immunity in many diseases where it is now clear that inflammation/immunity plays a critical role."

Also like her colleagues, Jouvin is still in the process of recruiting patients. As of November 2010, she had recruited only one. So if you want to volunteer, make contact!

Now bogies and bugs down in the dark of our gut just happens to be the topic of the next section too, forming a natural segue, as the disc jockeys like to call it!

Chapter 5 Our "Forgotten Organ"

If you are a health conscious individual and at all well read, you will know about Candida, also sometimes referred to as "yeast". It's been the buzzword for decades now.

> "This changed everything for me, about the way I viewed health and disease, and about the way I diagnosed and treated my patients.

I remember the excitement of reading first Orian Truss's two seminal papers in the Journal of Orthomolecular Psychiatry, back in 1978.

[Tissue injury induced by Candida albicans: Mental and neurologic manifestations. J. Ortho Psy, 7:1, 1978 and Restoration of Immunologic Competence to Candida Albicans. . J. Ortho Psy, 9:4, 1980 and The Role Of Candida Albicans in Human Illness, J. Ortho Psy, 10:4, 1981]

Dr. Truss is a psychiatrist from Birmingham, Alabama, with a special interest in clinical ecology; the study of how environmental factors affect health.

This changed everything for me, about the way I viewed health and disease, and about the way I diagnosed and treated my patients. Not that I mean Candida causes everything, as some seem to claim. But it certainly revealed an extensive and fascinating new area of personal investigation.

Truss introduced the catchy term "the missing diagnosis" and blamed Candida for a whole range of ills that were vague, difficult to identify or find a cause for and which were often written off as psychiatric in origin.

It's standard practice for impatient (and ignorant) doctors to blame the patient when he or she cannot find what's wrong. "It's all in your mind," is the standard and very unkind dismissive attitude of practitioners, even today.

Of course the real problem was that physicians were not looking in the right place, for the right cause, hence Truss's title: "the missing diagnosis".

The Problem Patient

Truss's work was taken up enthusiastically by the late Dr. William Crook, who did more than any single individual to popularize the Candida hypotheses, or what has now become known as 'the yeast connection', taken from the title of his book (*The Yeast Connection*, Professional Books, 1983)

Since that time, the whole theory seems to have gripped the public's imagination and clinical ecologists have been keen to extol the existence of the problem and the enormous benefits to be gained from tackling it vigorously. The fact is there are health gains to be made by following an anti-Candida program, taking antifungal drugs and excluding sugar and yeast foods from one's diet. Yet Truss's core idea remains no more than a theory.

If there is one valid complaint that members of the medical profession have against alternative practitioners, it is their tardiness in backing up ideas with research. It has been over three decades now since the first of Truss's innovative papers; ample time to carry out detailed studies that would validate his claims. Yet they are singularly lacking. A catalogue of startling recoveries does not constitute scientific study. We may be getting the right results for the wrong reason.

There are health gains to be made by following an anti-Candida program

Earlier Research

I started to look into this and search old published medical papers.

The deeper I probed, the more I found. Truss's ideas were anticipated almost 70 years earlier by a man called Turner, who presented a paper on what he called 'intestinal germ carbohydrate fermentation' (proceedings of the Royal Society of Medicine Symposium of Intestinal Toxaemia, 1911).

In 1931 Hurst was in his footsteps, writing about 'intestinal carbohydrate dyspepsia'. In the 1930s and 1940s this dyspepsia was being treated with Lactobacillus acidophilus, B vitamin supplements and a low-starch diet (remarkably like modern anti-Candida treatment except that legumes are no longer banned, as they were at that time).

Medical literature has tried to define the patient-type who suffers with this syndrome. A major text on gastroenterology in 1976 described victims as 'Essentially unhappy people . . . any suggested panacea or therapeutic straw is grasped. . . no regime is too severe and no program too difficult . . . with the tenacity of the faithful, they grope their way from one practitioner to the next in the search for a permanently successful remedy.'

The 'problem patient' attitude was probably what sank the condition in the 1950s. At that time, the psychosomatic theory of disease was enjoying a great revival. The tendency was to dismiss all patients with vague, ill-defined symptoms as psychiatric cases. Unlike today, there were no physical findings to disprove the psychiatric label and so it stuck. It's still with us, to a large degree.

Now, at last, we are starting to get some serious investigations and an amazing insight into what this is all about!

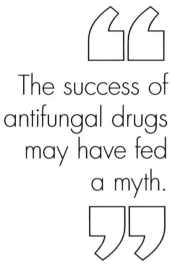

The success of antifungal drugs may have fed a myth.

Surgeons Who Blew Themselves Up!

The idea of a yeast-like organism that lives on starches and sugars and causes bowel disturbance is far from new then. It seems to enjoy a vogue in medical circles every few decades and then lapses out of sight once again. The reason is probably that, as in the 1980s, some doctors become convinced they know what causes the syndrome, but then can't seem to find a workable proof that affords a satisfactory explanation. This casts doubt on the basis of the theory. So it is today with 'Candida'.

The success of antifungal drugs may have fed a myth. In some cases, anti-Candida therapeutic agents such as Nystatin seem to work only in very high doses (10 to 100 times the usual dose). This has led to the speculation that it may be helping by some other mechanism than just that of eradicating the yeast micro-organism; possible by blocking bowel permeability.

One thing is certain, as I have already said: there is virtually no correlation between Candida in the stool sample and the existence of the 'yeast syndrome'. Indeed, Candida albicans is rarely identified in specimens, despite its known very wide occurrence. This lack of correlation is disappointing but hardly surprising, especially if we are looking for the wrong culprit.

It is true: treatment directed towards this type of organism can be highly effective in selected individuals, so clearly a real phenomenon exists. But that doesn't prove that Candida is to blame. In fact I'd like to set the debate alight with the claim that the culprit may not be Candida at all, or that Candida is only one of many potential suspects.

Other available flora that might be at work include the yeasts of the genus Saccharomyces (food yeasts), the bacteria Torulopsis glabrata and, most fascinating of all, Sarcina ventriculata.

Historically, Sarcina is an important organism. In the old days, when surgeons operated in frock coats and quite often smoked cigars at the same time, once in a while they would literally blow up their patients! As the alcoholic gases generated by Sarcina were released from the patient's stomach when cut open, the cigar would ignite the fumes and a fireball was the disastrous result. So literally: fire in the belly!

These 'on-board breweries' are probably quite common. Dr Keith Eaton called my attention to the speculation that so-called 'spontaneous combustion' may be due to this microbe. Puzzling cases have been documented of human beings literally vanishing in a sheet of fire, for no apparent reason. Perhaps Sarcina, or some other organism, and its inflammable gaseous excreta could be to blame.

I'm not going to do the whole "Candida" story of diagnosis and treatment here. I've summarized some of it in my own books *Diet Wise* and *The Moldy Patient*; the rest you can find in any number of books and postings online.

I hope merely, in the rest of this chapter, to persuade you that it's not NEARLY as simple as diagnosing Candida and going on a so-called "antifungal" diet. If you think dysbiosis and probiotics are just about Candida and taking yogurt, you've not understood! Dysbiosis is an exploding modern science with genetic and health implications for us all.

The truth is the full picture is a lot bigger and more amazing (frankly), than I or my colleagues could ever have guessed in those early years. Intelligent focus is now on a far bigger concept than just pathogens: I'm talking about the human microbiome.

The Human Microbiome

More fancy Greek: it just means the genetic make up of the bacteria and other microbes which live on us and in us. In fact 10% of our dry body weight is made up of bacteria. They have trillions of genes, compared to our measly few thousand.

Let's start with an understanding of the way it should be, before we look at pathological changes.

The fact is, we live in a sea of bacteria and other microbes. Not only that, but our bodies are inhabited by an on-board crowded colony of bacteria and other microbial life forms, such as viruses, archea (like early bacteria), fungi, yeasts, protozoa and parasites.

Our bodies have been likened to a coral reef! Science writer Ed Young calls us "Humanville", where hundreds of trillions of denizens reside.

We are born free of organisms, thanks to the sterile conditions in the womb. But it doesn't last. Within hours microbes contacted during birth jump on board (if you have ever attended a birth, you'll know how very UN-hygienic the process is!)

In fact mother's gift at birth, the sweat, urine, vaginal secretions and (can I say this?)… shit, is far from a problem and far from "one of those things". *It turns out to be absolutely vital to the child's healthy growth and development.*

Without this "transplant" of filth (OK, I'm just having fun painting this picture), the child would not grow up normally; its nervous system would be faulty and uneducated; even nervous system function would be severely compromised. Fortunately, babies born by Caesar get their "dose" from the surgical operatives and subsequent handling.

We've come a long way from the belief that microbes were a challenge to the infant, to realizing that it's very important for the newborn to meet them and get acquainted. The arrogance of science has had to give away to the humbling discovery that Nature knows more than we do and that we should follow Her process, not try to invent one of our own.

The Statistics

I already shared in my book *How To Survive In A World Without Antibiotics* that our dry body weight (minus all the water) is an amazing 10% bacteria and pathogens.

In fact, once grown, the average person is home to about 100 trillion microbes and they are everywhere, colonizing your gut, mouth, skin, mucous membranes and genitals. As science writer Claire Ainsworth put it, "you are born 100 per cent human, but die 90 per cent microbial. "

The combined genetic content of this vast colony of organisms we have started to view as a whole and entire: we call it the microbiome (like the human "genome", but for microbes). It might at first sight look like a bad idea to lump all these genes together. But in fact there are compelling reasons for doing so, which I shall come to.

By age 3, the mature human microbiome is in place, with the majority of microbes residing in the colon. Each of us carries hundreds of species from a total possible repertoire of more than 1000 different microbes (Nature, vol 464, p 59).

A new study shows that the abundance of certain bacterial genes in your feces correlates with your age, sex, body mass index and nationality. Increasing age, for example, is associated with an increase in the genes for enzymes needed to break down starches in the diet. Men seem to have more biochemical pathways for the synthesis of the amino acid aspartate than women. The microbiomes of overweight people (higher BMIs) were richer in genes involved in harvesting energy from gut contents. And people from different countries had small subsets of genes associated with their nationality (Nature, DOI: 10.1038/nature09944).

However, many microbial species are shared by us all, and the latest findings suggest that the overall ecological composition of microbes in any human gut falls into one of three basic groups, or "enterotypes" (Nature, DOI: 10.1038/nature09944).

> Increasing age, for example, is associated with an increase in the genes for enzymes needed to break down starches in the diet.

What They Do For Us

They don't just sit there! These microbes interact with us very beneficially. A balanced and healthy gut flora helps keep disease-causing microbes at bay by occupying their preferred niches.

In a normal gut of a lean individual, bacteria generally do more good than harm. Gut bacteria actively supplement our metabolism. The indigestible leftovers of our diet serve as the major food source for these resident bacteria, the greatest numbers of which reside in the distal gut, or large intestine.

They metabolize many dietary fibers that escape host digestion, generating short-chain fatty acids such as acetic, propionic, and butyric acids. These metabolites contribute an estimated 10 percent of our daily energy supply.

[Fukata M, Chen A, Vamadevan AS, Cohen J, Breglio K, Krishnareddy S, Hsu D, Xu R, Harpaz N, Dannenberg AJ, Subbaramaiah K, Cooper HS, Itzkowitz SH, Abreu MT: Toll-like receptor-4 promotes the development of colitis-associated colorectal tumors. Gastroenterology. 2007, 133:1869–81]

The amount and variety of these energy compounds produced are determined by the types of food ingested, how long the food stays in the gut, and which microbial species are present. While humans have the capacity to synthesize some short-chain fatty acids, the vast majority are produced by gut microbes. So we need our microflora.

The Butyrate Paradox

Butyric acid and related compounds in the colon (butyrates) are somewhat confusing, in that butyric acid is pretty obnoxious (it's used, for example, in "acid attacks" on abortion clinics by pro-life anti-abortionists), yet is seems to be a very powerful anti-inflammatory in the gut and is a valuable quencher of "fire in the belly".

Butyrate possesses both preventive and therapeutic potential to counteract inflammation-mediated ulcerative colitis (UC) and colorectal cancer.

Butyric acid seems to have a complex role in soothing the intestinal mucosa (gut lining). It actually feeds *colonocytes*, that is the cells lining the large bowel. It helps transport of nutrients from the bowel to the blood.

Without butyrates for energy, colon cells undergo autophagy (self digestion) and die.

[Donohoe, Dallas R.; Garge, Nikhil; Zhang, Xinxin; Sun, Wei; O'Connell, Thomas M.; Bunger, Maureen K.; Bultman, Scott J. (2011). "The Microbiome and Butyrate Regulate Energy Metabolism and Autophagy in the Mammalian Colon". Cell Metabolism 13 (5): 517–26. doi:10.1016/j.cmet.2011.02.018. PMC 3099420. PMID 21531334]

Butyrates reduce oxidation stress, meaning they act as a pretty good anti-oxidant. They also works as a barrier against leaky gut.

And if that's not enough, it increases satiety—meaning it gives you that full, not-hungry feeling.

[Aliment Pharmacol Ther. 2008 Jan 15;27(2):104-19. Epub 2007 Oct 25]

So, in principle, butyrates are probably beneficial, although there is still some argument. So where do we get them?

Short-chain fatty acids, which include butyrates, are produced by beneficial colonic bacteria (probiotics) that feed on, or ferment prebiotics, which are plant products that contain adequate amounts of dietary fiber.

[http://www.ncbi.nlm.nih.gov/pubmed/22517765]

Butyrate is a major metabolite in colonic lumen arising from bacterial fermentation of dietary fiber and has been shown to be a critical mediator of the colonic inflammatory response.

Acetates: it has been shown that microbial-generated acetate binds a receptor called GPR43, found on immune cells. Deletion of this receptor in mice exacerbated arthritis, asthma, and colitis—diseases characterized by an overactive immune system.

In other words, the microbially-produced acetate, as well as butyrate, may help steer inflammatory responses to a resolution. No wonder, then, that knocking out our healthy flora can lead to the massive widespread inflammation I have christened "Fire In The Belly"!

[Fukata M, Shang L, Santaolalla R, Sotolongo J, Pastorini C, España C, Ungaro R, Harpaz N, Cooper HS, Elson G, Kosco-Vilbois M, Zaias J, Perez MT, Mayer L, Vamadevan AS, Lira SA, Abreu MT: Constitutive activation of epithelial TLR4 augments inflammatory responses to mucosal injury and drives colitis-associated tumorigenesis. Inflamm Bowel Dis. 2010, [Epub ahead of print].

Premature babies, who do not get their inoculation of healthy pathogens at birth, since they are kept in strict hygienic conditions, are prone to a deadly bowel condition called necrotising enterocolitis. It kills up to 1 in 5 preemies. Doctors have failed to blame it on any one organism: it is probably due instead to the lack of protective fermentation products, such as butyrates and acetates, caused by a widespread reduction in micriobiota presence.

Gut Organisms Educate Us!

But it's more than that even. Gut flora are also involved in the development of the immune system. The gut, being technically "outside" the body, as I explained, is permanently in direct contact with our germ-infested everyday environment.

The immune system in the gut (Peyer's patches, etc.) becomes educated by sampling the gut flora. In mice kept sterile of microbes, immune tissue fails to mature properly and carries fewer of the signaling molecules that sense and react to pathogens.

Microbes also help in the formation of gut structure. The tiny little "hairs" we use for absorption called villi depend on our normal population of microbes for their formation. Villi develop abnormally in microbe-free mice.

But perhaps most startling of all: our gut microbes help with valuable neurological development. We now understand something called the gut-brain axis (remember the words of Phillipe Pinel in the opening paragraphs). It was there all the time and even appears in our language: from "gut feelings" to "having some guts", English is full of phrases where our bowels exert an influence upon our behavior. There are open lines of communication between brains and bowels and, in animal tests at least, these channels allow an individual's gut bacteria to steer their behavior.

The bacterial passengers of HMS Baby don't just react as their vessel develops; they help to steer it too. By studying mice, Rochellys Diaz Heijtz from the Karolinska Institute has found that a mammal's gut bacteria can affect the way its brain develops as it grows up. They could even influence how it behaves as an adult.

Under their influence, a baby's nerves will grow and connect in ways that will affect everything from how anxious to how coordinated it is. Thanks to that "messy" birth, an infant's brain is being shaped correctly by its gut.

> Our microbiome, it transpires, affects chronic diseases and the likelihood of obesity.

A New Organ

Our colony of onboard microbial passengers is such a large entity and so influential on our health, it has been likened to an extra organ, like a liver, heart or lungs. It's the unseen force that regulates how we process food, regulate our defenses against pathogens, and keep working like a healthy, well-oiled machine.

Our microbiome, it transpires, affects chronic diseases and the likelihood of obesity. They are essential to our digestion, by breaking down chemicals in our food that we wouldn't normally be able to process.

I have already explained in chapter 1 (page 14) that, with our new understanding of genomics, we know that humans have many tiny variations in gene sequencing called single nucleotide polymorphisms or SNPs (we usually say "snips"). From this we can say that everyone's ability to handle and metabolize food is different and probably unique. Therefore problems like food allergies and intolerance could be predicted, rather than scoffed at, as my enemies did in decades gone by. I was right!

Also, as I explained earlier, it becomes immensely more complicated when we grasp that the genes and SNPs of our onboard microbes also, as it turns out, can influence our tolerance of foods. Now you know why, when we clear up "Candida" or "yeasts" (far too simple a concept today), then our digestion and food tolerances improve dramatically.

The human microbiome influences our food sensitivities as much as our own immune system does! Wow!

Just how big is this? Well, it emerges our gut flora may even influence our sexual preferences! It's not certain yet with humans but studies by Gil Sharon at Tel Aviv University with the fruit fly showed clearly that the flies' sexual preferences change dramatically when they were fed antibiotics. So be warned.

Each microbiome is very distinctive. It turns out that we can identify a species, or even an individual, from the genetic makeup of these colonies. It's as individual as your passport or driving license! (Nature, DOI: 10.1038/nature09944).

No wonder then that blasting it all to hell with broad-spectrum antibiotics is a disaster. Health is about balance; once you upset the balance, total health is gone for good, unless you can somehow restore that balance.

Suddenly, dysbiosis (not a medially accepted term, by the way, but real nonetheless) starts to look like a dangerous condition.

See how much bigger this is than supposed "Candida"?

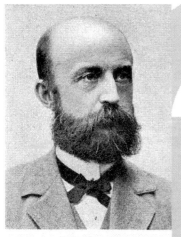

E. B. Almquist.

In 1922, Ernst Almquist, a colleague of Louis Pasteur, stated:

> Nobody can pretend to know the complete life cycle and all the varieties of even a single bacterial species. It would be an assumption to think so.

[Mattman LH. Cell Wall Deficient Forms: Stealth Pathogens: CRC Press; 2000]

While Almquist was never as recognized as Pasteur, his work on idiopathic bacteria in chronic disease readily foresaw the complexity that would later be inherent to the field of metagenomics and the human microbiome.

Let's Talk About Shit

Technically it's called faeces (feces, American spelling), after the Greek word for same. Call it poop, pooh, dung, dirt, crap, turds, whatever… We have to be frank and open here. Coyness is not scientific. Just turn your iPad or tablet to one side if you are reading this in a coffee shop!

You can tell a lot about a person's health from their pooh. In the old days, when people used a commode at night, it was great for doctors, who just asked to see what was produced!

Even with flush toilets, you can get clues.

Color: pale yellow means not enough bile getting through (bile digests into the brown color)

Identifiable food residues (other than just beet color and tomato skins) means incomplete digestive enzymes

Floating in the pan and sticking to the sides means there is fat still present. It should have digested out and so that, in turn, says there is not enough bile (which emulsifies fats) and not enough fat digestive enzymes (lipase); both liver and pancreas are implicated.

One of the biggest clues to bowel condition is the texture. What has emerged, thanks largely to the work of English surgeon Denis Burkett in Africa, that a large mushy pad like a cowpat is best. We don't much defaecate on the ground now, not in the West. But you can recognize this, even in a flush toilet. What you want is bulky, soft stools, which don't float, with a suitable dark color.

You do not want the constipated, dried rocks that are so typical of the average Westerner. It denotes lack of fiber and fiber, it has emerged, is crucial.

I used to joke that if that's all it was about, we could just chop up the carpets and eat those. Well, I have had to eat crow because it is NOT "just about fiber"; it's about fermented fiber and that's down to our old friends the microbiota population.

Flatulence, Farting, Blowing Off

While we are on about this, let me cover farting, though strictly speaking, it has little to do with what I'm calling Fire In The Belly. It's not something we talk about normally, the smell is an embarrassment and in certain situations, it can cause hilarity (remember the lift scene with Peter Sellers in the Revenge Of The Pink Panther movie: see it on YouTube if you have the patience to type in the correct address: http://www.youtube.com/watch?v=1TtZgs8k8dU).

The technical word flatulence comes from the Latin: *flatus*, a blowing. The word farting comes from our English-Germanic roots of our language; Anglo-Saxon *ferzen*, meaning the same thing.

But, as we all know, flatulence can relate to the health of the bowel and smelly, unhealthy farting is a possible indicator of dysbiosis.

Bloating is caused by gas in the intestine, mainly the colon. If the gas becomes excessive, flatulence results. It can come and go very dramatically. I have seen patients during a food challenge test enlarge their waistline in a matter of one or two minutes, putting on as much as 8 in/20 cm.

There seem to be certain food groups notoriously associated with flatulence: the pulses are notorious, beans and wind often being the subject of crude jokes; brassicas (cabbage, cauliflower, kale etc.) are not as widely recognized but are just as much trouble. Remember, it is not necessarily every member of a food family that causes a reaction.

Gluten enteropathy, or celiac disease, has long been associated with bloating, flatulence and bulky, stinking stools – indeed, these are important diagnostic signs.

Lastly, dysbiosis or intestinal fermentation syndrome can be very smelly, not associated with any particular food group.

The 4-letter "S" word

(Shit), there, I said it…

Scientists have been taking an unusual interest in pooh lately. Raw sewage contains thousands of undiscovered viruses, some of which could affect human health, a new study suggests.

Viruses are everywhere, meaning widespread, but only about 3,000 distinct viruses have been identified worldwide (surprisingly few).

In this study, researchers looked for the genetic signatures of viruses present in raw sewage in North America, Europe and Africa. They detected traces of 234 known viruses representing 26 different virus families, which makes raw sewage home to the most diverse collection of viruses ever documented.

Known viruses detected in raw sewage included human pathogens such as human papillomavirus, which can cause genital warts and cervical cancer, and norovirus, which causes stomach flu. There were also viruses associated with rodents and cockroaches, viruses from plants and viruses that prey on bacteria.

Most of the genetic signatures belonged to unknown viruses, many of which play unknown roles in human health and environmental processes. So there is even more to add to our "forgotten organ", the human microbiome. It's likely that many more viruses will come into view, now this new source has been discovered and looked at.

I think viruses found in the ocean are going to top raw sewage by orders of magnitude, although viruses won't be found in such densities as they are in sewage. The future awaits.

[journal BioMed, Oct 4, 2011]

71

Chapter 6 Smoldering Viruses

You have just read that our bowel flora and its microbiome include many viruses. Here is a section designed to extend your knowledge of this little-understood phenomenon.

> **"Is it not that we get the viruses because the immune system is poor or incompetent, rather than we get the immune dysfunction because of the virus?**

In the 1970s we started speaking about "smouldering viruses" (I lived in the UK then, so spelled it that way!); also sometimes referred to as "slow viruses". This meant sub-clinical virus opportunists that get under the radar of the immune system and can't be dislodged.

Instead, they hang on and linger, often for the entire lifetime of infected individuals, setting up chronic, damaging inflammation throughout the body. Diseases of aging and autoimmunity, and many other deadly ailments have been linked to such chronic stealth infections.

Once again, it was the clinical ecologists and alternative community who first spotted what was going on. We were open to think laterally and outside the box.

We started to talk about "post-viral fatigue syndrome", since the debility would not go away after the acute infectious episode. Fibromyalgia (ME in Europe) is typical of the pattern of symptoms for post-viral syndrome. Attention to allergies and intolerance often aided recovery a great deal. This pointed to a disordered immune response. But in my 1988 book *The Allergy Handbook*, I began asking "Is it not that we get the viruses because the immune system is poor or incompetent, rather than we get the immune dysfunction because of the virus?" I started thinking along the lines that environmental toxins debilitate the immune system, which then leads to the stealth virus. I have not been proved wrong. We just don't know.

Since those early years, so-called stealth-adapted viruses have been recovered from multiple tissues, including blood, cerebrospinal fluid, urine, throat swabs, breast milk, brain biopsies and tumor samples from patients with various neurological, psychiatric, auto-immune, allergic and cancerous diseases.

So this is a serious issue. And it is not confined to viruses.

Examples of neurological illnesses which could have this sort of basis include autism, attention deficit and behavioral disorders in children; depression, schizophrenia, amyotrophic lateral sclerosis (Lou Gehrig), multiple sclerosis, chronic fatigue and fibromyalgia in adults; and neurodegenerative illnesses in the elderly, such as Shy-Drager and multiple system atrophy.

Examples of the guilty viruses, which turn up time and time again, are Epstein-Barr virus, Coxsackie, cytomegalovirus, enterovirus and herpes viruses, notably human herpes virus 6 (HHV-6). Other organisms include mycoplasma, and bacteria, such as Chalamydia pneumoniae (Cpn) and Borrelia bugdorferii (true Lyme disease).

By following individual patients over several years, it has been found that there may be lateral transfer, leading to related but diverse illnesses within a family. Even pets may be affected.

The strange bone disorder called Paget's disease is now recognized as a "slow" version of the canine distemper virus. The actual disease emerges decades after the initial infection.

Community-wide outbreaks of stealth virus infections have also been observed with individuals showing varying levels of severity and duration of illness. This may be the cause of otherwise unexplainable deaths, and a strange "dumbing" of a whole township, as reflected in the excessive need for special education for its children.

The latter isn't surprising; it is now known that the stealth viruses can infect almost any organ, but that the brain is especially prone to manifest the effects of even limited localized cellular damage. If this is mixed in with an autoimmune response, the results can be complex and a diagnostic nightmare.

Indeed, I sometimes speculate that the current autism "epidemic" may be due to a stealth virus, as yet undiscovered. Or maybe a mutant version of the measles virus, from the vaccine, which is being spread among the population by mass use of the MMR vaccine.

Of course it is not politically correct to impugn vaccination. But there will be no answer to the autism riddle, till someone asks the right question.

Cancer can now be added to the list of potential stealth virus-associated diseases. The original of this was Burkitt's lymphoma, named after Denis Burkitt, who discovered it in Africa. Since then, more and more cancers are turning out to be mediated by viruses, including multiple myeloma and, more famously, cervical cancer, from the human papilloma virus (HPV).

A previous history of chronic fatigue in a cancer patient may provide a clue to loss of brain function, suggestive of an underlying

Community-wide outbreaks of stealth virus infections have also been observed with individuals showing varying levels of severity and duration of illness.

stealth virus infection in a cancer patient. It will be interesting to determine the effect of stealth-virus suppressive therapy in such patients. At this time such therapy is not being practiced.

However, preliminary research on mice shows the use of a vaccine against the common cold may have anti-cancer possibilities. This is ironic and relevant; the virus gets into the cancer cell, which allows it to hide from the immune system, and so the virus replicates and kills the host (cancer) cells. So the cold virus is being a "stealth virus" inside the cancer!

Finally, know that a stealth virus uses a novel strategy for replication. It has the capacity to "capture, amplify and mutate" genetic sequences assimilated from infected cells, other viruses and bacteria.

Don't forget that these "stealth pathogens" also form a part of the troublesome human microbiome, when we come to that. So this messing around with genes is a particularly troublesome aspect of this sneaky infectious nightmare.

Unfortunately, there are no reliable tests to date and stealth pathogens are notorious for imitating other organisms, so their true nature goes often unidentified. This makes them especially difficult to even study, never mind eliminate.

Be afraid; be very afraid, as the movie trailers say… moo-ha-ha-ha-ha!

Beyond The Slow Virus Theory

We now have a major new component of the stealth virus model; one which promises to yield powerful new healing modalities in the future.

It's the hypothesis by Dr. Hanan Polansky that fragments of foreign DNA from entrenched viruses can be very disruptive and dangerous. We've always known that viruses are basically just DNA. But it seems this foreign DNA doesn't have to even be viable to cause trouble. Even broken or damaged chunks of viral DNA can lead to chronic disease and inflammation.

Polansky calls these critical fragments of DNA "N-boxes". When foreign N-boxes enter the body (naturally, or artificially, like through an injection of some treatment, such as a vaccine), they end up in the nucleus of our cells, where they attract scarce genetic resources.

It is interesting that most common stealth viruses have strong N-boxes in their DNA. They include the Epstein-Barr virus (EBV), Cytomegalovirus (CMV), Herpes Simplex virus (HSV), Varicella Zoster virus (VZV), Hepatitis B Virus (HBV), Hepatitis C Virus (HCV), Human Papillomavirus (HPV), and others. In fact, the CMV virus has the strongest N-box known to science. This N-box is so strong that human genes cannot compete with its power to attract the scarce genetic resources.

The effect of competition for genetic resources is like the effect of a magnet. CMV is simply a very powerful magnet. It attracts away needed human material. The result? Our cells are starved for their own DNA processes!

It's like having bad genes, because the good genes can't function as they should. The viral DNA fragments are, in effect, genetic parasites.

We call this the "starved gene" model. Nice theory and its gathering ground. (See review comments at http://www.gene-eden.com/comments.htm)

Polansky coined the term "microcompetition". In the nucleus, this microcompetition between the foreign N-boxes and the human N-boxes in the human genes can, logically, lead to a great variety of diseases, where gene expression is at least a part of the picture. This works against us, apparently, even if the virus is very latent (inactive) or even if the viral DNA is broken into pieces and cannot express proteins.

I hope the theory bears up to full scrutiny, because Polansky's discovery has important implications. It suggests that we can cure and even prevent major diseases by targeting the foreign DNA fragments in the human body.

Is Obesity A Virus?

I found one interesting study on obesity, which tends to bear up Polansky's research and will be of interest to readers of "Fire In The Belly".

According to this recent longitudinal study in children, published in the Archives of Disease in Childhood, inactivity does not lead to fatness!

They found that, while body fat percentage was predictive of changes in physical activity over the following 3 years, physical activity levels were not predictive of subsequent changes in body fat.

Thus, while a 10% higher body fat at age 7 years predicted a relative decrease in daily moderate and vigorous intensities of 4 min from age 7 to 10 years, greater physical activity at 7 years did not predict a relative decrease in body fat between 7 and 10 years.

The authors therefore concluded that the known association between lower activity levels and higher body fat may be the result of fatness leading to inactivity rather than inactivity driving body fat. In other words, physical inactivity appears to be the result of fatness rather than its cause.

[Metcalf BS, Hosking J, Jeffery AN, Voss LD, Henley W, & Wilkin TJ (2010). Fatness leads to inactivity, but inactivity does not lead to fatness: a longitudinal study in children (EarlyBird 45). Archives of disease in childhood PMID: 20573741]

On Polasnky's model, one of the causes of obesity is an infection with a stealth virus.

The cause of obesity is not lack of activity, and it's not necessarily "bad" eating habits!

The microcompetition for DNA resources "starves" the human genes and forces them to behave as if they've been mutated, that is, to behave as if they are dysfunctional and therefore cannot stop fat cells from multiplying and accumulating fat.

You might be interested in Polansky's patented formula for eliminating stealth viruses. It's called Gene-Eden. To develop Gene-Eden, the scientists at polyDNA analyzed thousands of papers and identified the most effective and safe antiviral natural ingredients.

Just always bear in mind my maxim: *beware the science from someone who is trying to sell you something!* It applies in alternative health, just as much as Big Pharma and commerce in general.

For a free copy Dr. Polansky's book, visit http://www.cbcd.net and click on free download. For more information on Gene-Eden, visit http://www.Gene-Eden.com. A word of warning though: it's very heavy reading indeed.

The cause of obesity is not lack of activity, and it's not necessarily "bad" eating habits!

Metagenomics

Looking further at the vast collection of DNA and genes we carry, it soon becomes obvious why all this is important.

For one thing, many species cannot be grown in the lab. The only way we have been able to find them is because of their DNA imprint.

The ability to extract DNA directly from samples and sequence it spawned a wealth of studies that build a picture of what is living inside us. Most of it is bacteria; a tiny minority of the flora are fungi and protozoa, about which little is known. The same goes for the viruses that lurk in the gut, preying on the bacteria there. These seem to comprise mostly unknown species and vary hugely from one individual to another (Nature, vol 466, p 334).

All this is being extensively studied by Metagenomics of the Human Intestinal Tract (MetaHIT), a European Union-based consortium. The researchers studied fecal samples taken from 124 European adults and found a staggering 3.3 million different microbial genes, meaning that they outnumber our own human gene set about 150-fold (Nature, vol 464, p 59).

We are then, in effect, a sort of combined "super-organism" that functions as a whole which is more than just its parts.

The team has identified a set of genes we all share. It's capable of more than six thousand biochemical functions and represents the core genes needed for the survival of the entire ecosystem that is a human being.

So what do these genes do? Many seem to be plugging metabolic gaps in our own genome. It is common knowledge that we are unable to synthesize enough vitamin B or any vitamin K without our gut flora, but microbes assume many other useful functions.

For example, they contain genes that convert complex carbohydrates into simpler molecules called short-chain fatty acids, an important energy source accounting for between 5 and 15 per cent of our requirements.

Other core genes break down plant cellulose and complex sugars such as pectin, found in fruit and vegetables, which allows us to digest foods we could not handle without them.

The MetaHIT project also found microbial genes that seem to be involved in metabolizing drugs and other non-dietary compounds, such as toxins and food additives.

So this is an entirely new twist on chemical sensitivity. It also fits entirely with my clinical observations, which I published decades ago: that "Candida" or dysbiosis cases were usually extremely chemically sensitive (part of my "awesome foursome" syndrome, indicating dysbiosis).

So, "personalized" medicine just became vastly more complicated. This is an indirect inflammation, caused by a disordered microbiome.

A Note About "Natural" Antibiotics

We all like the idea of using natural plant, animal and fungal sources as antibiotics. Some of these are great. I published scores of such remedies, with good science to back them up, in my important book How To Survive In A World Without Antibiotics (www.MRSAhotline.com)

But it would naïve to assume that so-called natural antibiotic substances will not harm our microbiome. There is no rationale for such a belief. Some of them almost certainly would damage it. I'm thinking of hydrogen peroxide and MMS (chlorine dioxide protocol), for instance.

There is absolutely no science on this point and, until there is, I suggest due caution with all supposed natural remedies.

When It Goes Wrong

So now we are beginning to get a much more technical and understandable view of what "dysbiosis" is really all about and why it is such a disaster.

A study published recently showed that gut flora composition alters dramatically in response to a course of antibiotics, before starting to rebuild itself after about a week (Proceedings of the National Academy of Sciences, vol 108, p 4554). "It does mostly bounce back but certainly not quite all the way," says Les Dethlefsen from Stanford University in California, one of the research team. He speculates that repeated disturbances of the ecological balance of the gut microbiome could permanently shift the functioning of the ecosystem - an alteration that would then be passed down from parent to child. "Every time we perturb the community, there is a roll of the dice," he says.

Among the participants in the MetaHIT project was a group of people with inflammatory bowel diseases such as ulcerative colitis and Crohn's disease. Previous research suggested that this group would have a lower diversity of bacterial species in their guts; that's a natural after-effect of frequent antibiotic use.

It follows, therefore, that they have fewer microbial genes. Sure enough, those in the MetaHIT study had 25 per cent less than healthy people.

Meanwhile, research in mice indicates that the balance of microbes in the gut can play a part in the development of type 2 diabetes. People with the disease harbour a greater proportion of Bacteroidetes bacteria than Firmicutes, according to research published last year (PLos One, vol 5, p e9085). That would go some way to explain the current "epidemic" of diabetes; it follows in the wake of excess antibiotic use and food contamination with antibiotics.

Gut flora might also be associated with obesity; another twist of the story I have with Hanan Polansky's work. When a team led by Jeffrey Gordon from Washington University in St Louis took microbes from the guts of lean and obese mice and transplanted them into germ-free mice, they found that those with the microbiome of obese mice put on significantly more weight (Nature, vol 444, p 1027). Subsequent studies indicate that the microbiomes of obese humans have a greater ability to harvest energy from food (Obesity, vol 18, p 190).

Research in mice indicates that the balance of microbes in the gut can play a part in the development of type 2 diabetes.

Inflammatory Dangerous "Belly Fat"

People store body fat in two main ways:

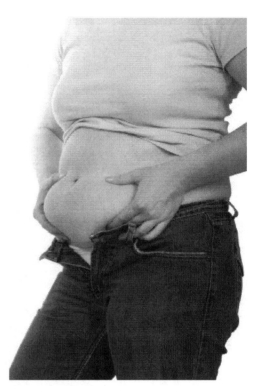

- Just under the skin in the thighs, hips, buttocks, and abdomen. That's called subcutaneous fat.

- Deeper inside, around the vital organs (heart, lungs, digestive tract, liver, etc.) in the chest, abdomen, and pelvis. That's called visceral fat or more casually "belly fat", since it sticks out most in the abdomen.

Subcutaneous fat is the fat we can see, and visceral fat is the fat we can't.

Fat doesn't just sit idle. It acts like an organ that secretes substances. Even worse, it holds onto toxic compounds, like pesticides and other pollutants and can release them over time. Having a preponderance of belly fat means you are more likely to suffer inflammation from pollutants and more likely to have a heart attack or stroke (which are mainly inflammatory processes, anyway).

It has been shown that inflammatory compounds released by visceral fat cells can also lead to insulin resistance and some cancers. Excess visceral fat is also linked to greater risk of high blood pressure, type 2 diabetes, heart disease, dementia, and cancers of the breast, colon, and endometrium.

Again these are inflammatory diseases in nature or with a strong inflammatory component (like cancer).

Where your body stores fat depends on your genes, lifestyle factors (such as stress and whether you get enough sleep), age, and sex.

Men under 40 tend to have a higher proportion of visceral fat to subcutaneous fat than women. Women store more visceral fat after menopause.

In an obese person, the body can run out of safe places to store fat and begin storing it in and around the organs, such as the heart and the liver.

Non-alcoholic fatty liver disease (NAFLD) was once rare. But with obesity increasing, it occurs more and more. NAFLD causes more cirrhosis than alcohol abuse, so this is a critical subject.

Measuring Your Fat Load

CT scan or MRI is the most precise way to see where fat is stored. But there are simple – and free -- calculations that can show how you might be storing your fat.

Most experts agree that, no matter what your weight, a waist circumference over 35 inches for a woman and over 40 for a man indicates that you may have unsafe levels of visceral fat.

Measuring your waist sounds simple enough. But to make sure you get it right, here are instructions from the National Heart Lung and Blood Institute:

- Stand up. Exhale before you measure -- do not suck in your breath.

- Wrap the tape measure around your middle. It should go across your navel.

- Make sure bottom of the tape measure is just above your hip bones. It does not go higher up, even if you're narrower there.

While you're at it, measure your hips, too. Waist-to-hip ratio also indicates fat distribution. According to the Western Journal of Medicine, a healthy ratio is up to 0.8 for women and up to 0.9 for men. The journal offers these guidelines for an accurate hip measurement:

- Stand up. Place the tape measure around your hips.

- Make sure the tape goes over the knobby protrusions of the hip bones.

To get your waist-to-hip ratio, divide your waist measurement by your hip measurement.

BMI, Pears, and Apples

What about BMI? It relates your height to your weight. But it doesn't show where we're storing our fat. In fact it doesn't really help to identify obesity. According to BMI measurement, Michael Jordan, one of the US's greatest ever athletes, is obese!

Best forget about BMI. Put it this way:

Having a "pear shape," with fatter hips and thighs, is considered safer than the "apple shape," which describes a wider waistline.

Typically, if you are at a healthy weight, you'll have healthy levels of visceral fat, as well. But genes can predispose a person to being thin and still having a disproportionate amount of visceral fat.

Like overweight people with excess visceral fat, thin people with a genetic tendency to store visceral fat may have higher cholesterol and blood sugar due to insulin resistance.

So a thin person showing up with unusually high levels of cholesterol and blood sugar, may be the type who is storing visceral fat.

Importantly, an inactive lifestyle can also lead thin people to store fat viscerally, according to a study at the British Medical Research Council.

Reducing Inflammatory Visceral Fat

There are four key factors: exercise, diet, sleep, and stress management.

Exercise: No question staying active works. Vigorous aerobic exercise has been shown to trim subcutaneous and visceral fat, even fat stores in the liver linked to fatty liver disease. It's also proven to slow the build-up of visceral fat over the years.

In a Duke University study, 30 minutes of vigorous aerobic activity, done four times per week, reduced subcutaneous and visceral abdominal fat. Resistance training alone reduced only subcutaneous fat.

In this context, "vigorous" means jogging for physically fit people or walking briskly at an incline for obese people who may risk injury by jogging. Workouts of the same intensity on stationary bikes and elliptical or rowing machines are also effective.

Basically, raising your heart rate for 30 minutes at least three times per week – significantly slows visceral fat gain.

Diet: There is no diet that targets visceral fat alone. But when you lose weight, belly fat usually goes first.

A fiber-rich diet may help and has the bonus of working like a pre-biotic. People who eat 10 grams of soluble fiber per day, without any other diet changes, build up less visceral fat over time than others. That's two small apples, a cup of green peas, and a half-cup of pinto beans, for example.

Sleep: Too much or too little sleep also plays a role in the build-up of visceral fat. Lack of sleep, we know, is stressful and pro-inflammatory. A study published in Sleep tracked adults' visceral fat over five years. People who slept five hours or less, or eight or more hours, per night gained more visceral fat than those who slept between six and seven hours per night.

Stress: Managing your stress matters. That includes chronic stress you face in your personal life, and societal stresses. We can't always control stress but we can modify our response to it. Helpful factors include getting social support, meditating, and exercising as ways to handle stress.

Keeping up with your friends may also help. A study published in Biological Psychiatry showed that men and women who got support from a best friend before a stress test made less cortisol, the bad stress hormone. And another study, published in the International Journal of Psychiatry in Medicine, showed that women who pray or meditate have healthier levels of cortisol than those who don't meditate.

What if you only have time for one of these factors? Which one should you choose?

Exercize, without a doubt, is the key. It even beats dieting.

Is Fat A Communicable Disease?

There is now no question that genes play a part in the expression of obesity. The idea of an "obesity gene" is not silly. The question is: whose genes? Ours or the microbiomes?

The Dutch famine of 1944-1945 provides a unique opportunity to study humans exposed to well-defined under-nutrition. Adults who were exposed to poor nutrition in utero had an increased prevalence of glucose intolerance, dyslipidemia, early coronary heart disease, and obesity.

A recent study of adults who were exposed to the Dutch famine early in gestational development is reportedly the first to provide empiric support for the hypothesis that environmental exposures can cause epigenetic changes in humans.

[Roseboom T, de Rooij S, Painter R. The Dutch famine and its long-term consequences for adult health. Early Hum Dev 2006;82(8):485-91]

This in itself, is breakthrough science by the way. It was not supposed to happen—and cannot happen in the Darwinian

> I think the only logical conclusion is that GM foods will certainly set up inflammation, since we already know that normal foods do so.

evolution model; but it gives support to an older model: transmitted, acquired adult traits, as suggested by Frenchman Jean-Baptiste Lamarck (1744–1829)

Manipulating the microbiome could help manage weight. Bacteria in the intestine play a crucial role in digestion. They provide enzymes necessary for the uptake of many nutrients, synthesize certain vitamins and boost absorption of energy from food. Fifty years ago, farmers learned that by tweaking the microbial mix in their livestock with low-dose oral antibiotics, they could accelerate weight gain. Bad way to go but it does make the point.

You Are NOT what you eat, after all. Another myth bites the dust! What you eat counts—but your microbiota count more, it seems, meaning if you have the right microbiota, with the right genes, you can eat foods that will make others gain weight relentlessly.

The reverse is unpleasant: if you have the wrong microbiota, you will be overweight, no matter what you do. Losing weight will be a result of immense effort and will quickly revert to obesity, as soon as you take your eye off the ball. But it's even more depressing to realize you could eat exactly the same diet as a healthy, slim person, but you would gain weight on the same intake, calorie for calorie.

More recently, scientists found that mice raised in a germ-free environment, and thus lacking any gut microbes, do not put on extra weight, even on a high-fat diet.

In a study, published Aug. 26 2012 in the journal Nature Immunology, a research team based at the University of Chicago focused on the relationship between the immune system, gut bacteria, digestion and obesity. They showed how weight gain requires not just calories but also the wrong microbiota.

The interplay between intestinal microbes and the immune response proved just as important as the food intake.

According to the study's senior author Yang-Xin Fu, MD, PhD, professor of pathology at the University of Chicago Medicine, "Host digestion is not completely efficient, but changes in the gut flora can raise or lower digestive efficiency."

So the old adage "you are what you eat" needs to be modified to include, "as processed by the microbial community of the distal gut and as regulated by the immune system!"

To measure the effects of microbes and immunity, the researchers compared normal mice with mice that have a genetic defect that renders them unable to produce lymphotoxin, a molecule that helps to regulate interactions between the immune system and bacteria in the bowel. Mice lacking lymphotoxin, they found, do not gain extra weight, even after prolonged consumption of a high-fat diet.

On a standard diet, both groups of mice maintained a steady weight. But after nine weeks on a high-fat diet, the normal mice increased their weight by one-third, most of it fat. Mice lacking lymphotoxin ate just as much, but did not gain weight.

It is important to note that the high-fat diet triggered changes in gut microbes for both groups. The normal mice had a substantial increase in a class of bacteria (Erysopelotrichi) previously associated with obesity and related health problems. Mice that lacked lymphotoxin were unable to clear segmented filamentous bacteria, which has previously been found to induce certain immune responses in the gut.

To clinch it, the researchers transplanted bowel contents from the study mice to normal mice raised in a germ-free environment (without a microbiome, in other words). Mice who received commensal bacteria from donors that made lymphotoxin gained weight rapidly. Those that got the bacteria from mice lacking lymphotoxin gained much less weight for about three weeks, until their own intact immune system began to normalize their bacterial mix.

This is interesting too: when housed together, the mice performed their own microbial transplants. Mice are coprophagic; they eat each other's droppings. In this way, the authors note, mice housed together "colonize one another with their own microbial communities."

After weeks together, even mice with the immune defect began to gain weight. They also were able to reduce the presence of segmented filamentous bacteria in their stool.

[REFERENCE: Press release, Aug 27, 2012, University of Chicago]

Kissing Makes you Fat?

Is that saying even a person you kiss could infect you with weight gain microbes? In a way, yes! In fact it has been suggested that obesity is a kind of "communicable disease". I'm serious! Someone called it "Infectobesity"!

Bacteroides seem to be the pro-health bacteria and the firmiculites might not be so good. The % weight loss correlates to the ratio between bacteroides and firmiculites. Certainly the latter are better at extracting calories from food. Fiermiculites also activate enzymes that promote fat storage. Obese individuals have a ratio of 80% firmiculites to 20% bacteroides. Moreover, mice given low-fat, plant-based chow grew more bacteroides and less firmiculites and stayed lean

[presentation to the American College For The Advancement of Medicine, Nov 16 – 18, 2012, Las Vegas, Nevada, New Developments in Gut Health and It's Relationship To Systemic Illness]

In the last 2 decades at least 10 adipogenic (fattening) pathogens have been identified, associated with human obesity. These include viruses, scrapie agents, other bacteria and gut microflora.

The link between obesity and inflammation has also become very clear, so it's a bad story. You need to guard against this.

Stress comes into it. Mice subjected to social stress (2 hours a day for 6 days with an aggressive mouse) ended up with a significantly reduced bacteroides population, while increasing the more dangerous Clostridia species. There was also an increase in inflammatory cytokines and pre-treatment with antibiotics blocked this. So there is little doubt that the stressed microbiota were causing the inflammation.

This is all hot stuff, incredibly new and vital for the right lifestyle!

So Now, Of Course, Inflammation

Well, it's taken a long time to get here. But now I hope you will begin to sense the ENORMOUS influence of our gut flora for health. I now return you to Hippocrates' quote: all diseases begin in the intestine. He was not wrong, as you see.

Not only is bowel upset a huge potential source of inflammatory processes but also, more importantly, if our microbiome goes out of healthy adjustment, almost ANY disease can get started in its wake, from obesity to diabetes; heart disease to Alzheimer's and colitis to cancer.

The gut-brain axis I have referenced also does justice to Philipe Pinel's quote, also on page 2:

You will see why my chosen title "Fire In The Belly" was pretty apt (in a poetic , rather than scientific, sort of way).

Fecal Transplants and The Benefits Against Inflammation

You are now in a good position to understand another logical approach to the "Fire In The Belly" problem, which is turning out very well in clinical practice.

Now you realize the effects of a messed up intestinal flora, with missing healthy microbiome components and the presence of unwanted, dangerous and inflammatory fragments of foreign, unwelcome DNA, you will probably see that a good clean out and replacing the fouled up intestinal contents with healthier stuff is perhaps a good idea.

Strange as it may seem, some doctors are using this treatment. It's called a fecal microbiota transplant and it is helping diseases as diverse as colitis, auto-immune disorders and even Alzheimer's disease (which I have already commented is largely inflammatory in character).

Previous terms for the procedure include fecal bacteriotherapy, fecal transfusion, fecal transplant, stool transplant, fecal enema and human probiotic infusion (HPI).

A fecal microbiota transplant (FMT) involves restoration of the colonic flora by introducing normal bacterial flora through infusion of stool obtained from a healthy donor. It can also be used in other conditions apart from CDI including colitis, constipation, Irritable Bowel Syndrome and some neurological conditions, such as Alzheimer's disease

[Borody TJ, George L, Andrews P et al. Bowel-flora alteration: a potential cure for inflammatory bowel disease and irritable bowel syndrome? Med J Aust 1989; 150: 604].

It's a repulsive idea to many, though the semi-mystical healer known as Paracelsus (1493 –1541) actually administered fecal pellets as part of his protocols. He's always been admired by congoscenti of alternative healing.

Recently I learned that Theodor Morrell, Hitler's personal physician, was feeding the Fuehrer fecal pellets (along with other startling drugs, such as methamphetamines by injection). Presumably Herr H. didn't know that, otherwise it would have been the gas chamber for Morrell. But this occasional use has always been regarded as quackery and it's hard even for me to defend it.

In a sense, FMT is the ultimate quenching of the fire in the belly and the ultimate probiotic therapy!

FMT has been developed in more recent years by Dr Thomas J Borody and his team in Sydney, Australia, primarily as an alternative treatment for Clostridium difficile infection, including pseudomembranous colitis.

At the Centre for Digestive Diseases in Sydney, FMT is now being extended beyond CDI, to other conditions including ulcerative colitis, autoimmune disorders, neurological conditions, obesity and metabolic syndrome/diabetes.

The future of FMT is likely to move away from crude, homogenised human flora and progress towards the use of highly refined stool, comprising bacteria only, frozen and stored for usage. Ultimately such an extract can be dried, powdered and encapsulated to be administered as an enteric coated medication for use in a number of flora-related conditions [*Wikipedia* entry].

The Food Allergy Tie In With Genes and MicroRNA

Early on, I told you about the effects of small genetic variables, called single nucleotide polymorphisms.

I also said that changing foods can switch on good genes and switch off bad genes; a topic that we call epigenetics. With a fuller understanding of this process, it is easier to see why removing inflammatory and badly tolerated foods should have such a profound health effect.

How much more complicated it becomes, to realize that much of the genetic material in food survives digestion and circulates through the body, potentially setting up an inflammatory response. Often these food particles bind with antigens to form antigen-antibody complexes. These circulating "immune complexes" were well known to us clinical ecologists, as early as the start of the 1980s and seemed to be the origin of a particular type of food allergic response we called "delayed hypersensitivity reaction" or type IV immune response.

Indeed, I have always taught that naturally circulating foodstuffs, if you are reacting to it, will keep you permanently ill, till you stop eating the offending foods! The converse of that is that if you eliminate those foods, you will not only feel much healthier, but your immune system will be unburdened and able to function far better.

This could be the key reason why my patients with cancer did so extraordinarily well, defying all predictions by seeming to go on and on, without deteriorating, even though they had cancer.

Now these concepts are backed up and extended by new work, which has discovered that fragments of food RNA have been found swimming in the bloodstreams of people and cows. What's more the study by Chen-Yu Zhang of Nanjing University in China and his colleagues shows that some of these plant RNAs alter gene expression and raise cholesterol levels in mice. The discovery opens up a new way to turn food into medicine: we may be able to design plants that change our genes for the better.

This is such a big deal now that the cosmetic industry is on to it. Cosmetics researchers recently suggested that a pill containing a mix of food extracts can influence our genes and boost collagen production in the skin, reducing the appearance of wrinkles (New Scientist, 24 September, p 10).

Let's talk about GM crops

Do the genes firms insert into genetically modified crops change the health of people who eat them? We do not yet know the answer. But it is beginning to emerge they can cause inflammation and cancer.

What is clear is that the DNA of normal foods appears in the blood and the rest of our tissues. It would be impossible for regulators to deny that, therefore, DNA fragments of GM foods will be circulated throughout our tissues.

This violates the old assumption that food DNA is fully digested.

But it also means that GM foods are not intrinsically more dangerous than normal foods. If you search websites which oppose GM, they are quick to point out that GM fragments will get into our bloodstream but omit to mention that this happens to normal foods too (it would spoil their argument).

One particular study "On the fate of foreign DNA in mice" by Shubbert et al (1998) showed that ingested DNA from a bacterial virus is incorporated in chromosomes and is passed from mother to fetus. The authors of the study ask "is maternally ingested foreign DNA a potential mutagen for developing fetus?"

[Schubbert R, Hohlweg U, Renz D and Doerfler W (1998). "On the fate of orally ingested foreign DNA in mice: chromosomal association and placental transmission to the fetus" (1998) Mol Gen Genet 259: 569-576]

It's a reasonable question but, again, doesn't give GM foods a worse position than normal foods, which clearly can do so too.

I think the only logical conclusion is that GM foods will certainly set up inflammation, since we already know that normal foods do so. Therefore we must be cautious and take it food by food, crop by crop.

Thus, an important study led to the scrapping of a GM peas project in the last stages of its research, when it was learned that peas modified to resist insects had caused inflammation in the lung tissues of mice.

[Prescott VE, Campbell PM, Moore A and others (2005). Transgenic expression of bean alpha-amylase inhibitor in peas results in altered structure and immunogenicity. Journal of Agricultural and Food Chemistry 53(23):9023-9030.]

This at least was honest. Meantime, remain particularly wary of the shabby kind of science that seems to have entered the arena of safety testing for GMO foods, no doubt inspired by the mega-corporations like Monsanto (or MonSatan, as I heard it referred to once).

An example of the questionable research I am referring to is part of the Food Standards Agency (FSA) project on evaluating the risks of GMOs in human foods, commissioned by the former UK Ministry of Agriculture, Fisheries and Food (MAFF).

A single meal containing GM soya was fed to human subjects in the form of burgers and a soya protein supplement. No data were presented on how much DNA was present in the commercial samples, and whether the DNA was broken down and to what degree. Needless to say, the GM DNA inserts were not characterized at all.

The method of detecting GM DNA was highly flawed. It searched for a tiny fragment of the entire GM DNA insert that was at least ten or twenty times as long. So, any other fragment of the insert would not be detected. The chance of getting a positive result was thus 5% at best, and likely to be much, much less.

More revealing still, the researchers checked for GM DNA only in the gut contents, but failed to check if the DNA has passed through the gut into the blood stream and blood cells. This omission is inexcusable, as a series of experiments in mice dating back to 1997 had already documented that GM DNA can pass through the gut wall into the bloodstream, to be taken up by cells in the blood, liver and spleen.

When fed to pregnant mice, the GM DNA also passed through the placenta to be taken up by the cells of the fetus and the newborn.

[http://www.i-sis.org.uk/hgthumangut.php accessed online 6/3/2012, 10.48 am PST]

So beware of the science and avoid GM foods as best you can. But remember (as I keep saying) a carrot is a GM food; it was originally purple but the clever Dutch manipulated its genes to become its present color, in honor of their king, William of Orange!

Chapter 7 Inflammatory Bowel Disease

It's time we took a look at inflammation of the bowel itself. We call this inflammatory bowel disease and it covers several different but essentially similar pathologies, in which the intestines (small and large intestines) become inflamed (red and swollen).

This inflammation can cause a variety of symptoms such as:

- Severe or chronic (almost all of the time) pain in the abdomen (belly)
- Diarrhea — may be bloody
- Unexplained weight loss
- Loss of appetite
- Bleeding from the rectum
- Joint pain
- Skin problems
- Fever

Symptoms can come and go, sometimes going away for months or even years at a time. When people with IBD start to have symptoms again, they are said to be having a relapse or flare-up. When they are not having symptoms, the disease is said to have gone into remission.

The most common forms of IBD are ulcerative colitis and Crohn's disease (pronounced crones). The diseases are very similar. In fact, it's sometimes hard to figure out which type of IBD a person has. The main difference between the two diseases is the parts of the digestive tract they affect.

Ulcerative colitis affects the top layer of the large intestine, next to where the stool is. The disease causes swelling and tiny open sores, or ulcers, to form on the surface of the lining. The ulcers can bleed and produce pus. In severe cases of ulcerative colitis, ulcers may weaken the intestinal wall so much that a hole develops. Then the contents of the large intestine, including bacteria, spill into the abdominal (belly) cavity or leak into the blood. This causes a serious infection and requires emergency surgery.

Crohn's disease can affect all layers of the intestinal wall. Areas of the intestines most often affected are the last part of the small intestine, called the ileum, and the first part of the large intestine. But Crohn's disease can affect any part of the digestive tract, from the mouth to the anus. Inflammation in Crohn's disease often occurs in patches, with normal areas on either side of a diseased area.

In Crohn's disease, swelling and scar tissue can thicken the intestinal wall. This narrows the passageway for food that is being digested. The area of the intestine that has narrowed is called a stricture (STRIK-choor). Also, deep ulcers may turn into tunnels, called fistulas (FISS-choo-luhss), that connect different parts of the intestine. They may also connect to nearby organs, such as the bladder or vagina, or connect to the skin. And as with ulcerative colitis, ulcers may cause a hole to develop in the wall of the intestine.

Other Types Of Inflammatory Bowel Disease

These are not the only two inflammatory bowel disease. In fact food-borne infections may cause a transient inflammation but these are not usually counted.

You may have heard of, or be suffering from:

- Collagenous colitis

- Microscopic colitis (lymphocyte invasion of tissues, seen only under a microscope)

- Pseudomembranous colitis (caused by the organism C. difficile)

- Radiation-induced colitis (after exposure to radio-activity)

Note that irritable bowel syndrome (IBS) is different, though the symptoms can be similar. Unlike inflammatory bowel disease, it does not cause inflammation or damage in the intestines.

Mechanisms Predisposing IBD

- There is a genetic disposition, sure

- Food allergies and intolerance

- Leaky gut (page 43)

- Dysbiosis (unhealthy microbiome)

- Altered signalling or "cross-talk" between a healthy microbiome and enterocytes.

- Cytokine activation

The latter, in practice, is caused by all the other factors.

Stress and eating certain foods may not cause IBD. But both can make IBD symptoms worse.

Basically, IBD is an over-reaction or an unnecessarily prolonged reaction, when the inflammatory process just won't shut off. It no longer makes sense and is no longer relevant, no matter the initiating factors.

IBD runs in families. This suggests that inherited factors called genes play a role in causing IBD. Experts think that certain genes may cause the immune system to overreact in IBD.

But, as we have seen, genes can mean anything in this context: microbial genes could be to blame. We get out microbiota from our parents, principally mother, so whatever problem she has, we'll likely get.

Other Predisposing Factors

- "Western Diet" (American SAD diet)

- Excessive hygiene (no training for the immune system)

- Heredity

- Smoking cessation (yes, stopping smoking can bring it on, for reasons not really understood)

- Latitude (northern climates are worse)

- Dugs: proton pump inhibitors or PPIs, aspirin, NSAIDs

Other speculated factors include vaccination, milk consumption (I go for that one), appendicectomy or appendectomy if you can't spell (see page 47 on the real function of the appendix), stress, lack of breast feeding and SSRIs (remember most of our serotonin is in the gut, so SSRIs create too much. SSRI stands for selective serotonin reuptake inhibitors, meaning they cause an accumulate of serotonin by stopping its re-uptake and subsequent breakdown, after neuron firing).

An amusing one is toothpaste as a risk. This is something that still circulates and keeps coming up from time to time. I remember it mentioned even when I was a kid; it was supposed to allow sticky little particles to get stuck in the appendix, whence they caused trouble.

But then my biology teacher spouted quite a lot of what later turned out to be baloney!

Still, there are scientists that go for the evidence on this one: researchers state that they have found pigments in the intestinal mucosa containing aluminum, silicon, and titanium through electron microscopy and x-ray analytical techniques. In other studies, they have found not only toothpaste residues but traces of other materials used in dental work. They have suggested that further research be done on the role of toothpaste, food additives, and synthetic food ingredients as possible causative agents in inflammatory bowel disease.

Other particles that may be associated with gut inflammation include:

- Titanium dioxide (anatase) found in a lot of commercial vitamin formulas

- Mixed silicates

- Aluminosilicates

- Calcium phosphate (cement!)

- Anatase

- Soil residue

- Carrageenan (part of cosmetic testing)

- Titanium crystals are very sharp and, if present, would definitely set up pain and inflammation.

Conventional Treatments

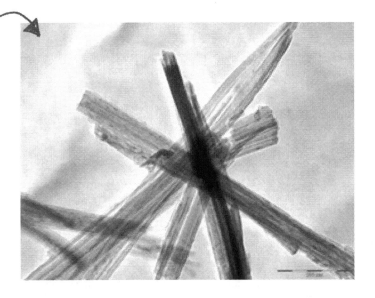

On the whole, orthodox treatments are unhelpful and may be damaging. Persistent reliance on just these therapies shows ineptness on the part of a gastroenterologist.

- Steroids

- Antibiotics

- Aminosalicylates

- Immuno-suppresive agents (mercaptopurine, methotrexate and the like – chemotherapy, in other words)

- Biologics (Anti tumor necrosis factor alpha (TNF-alpha), therapies have been used for years to treat Crohn's disease and are now being used for ulcerative colitis)

- Surgical resection (bad call, surgeons often end up taking away more and more intestine, in a desperate but vain effort to prevent recurrence)

- Total colectomy and a colostomy bag (the end of the line, after all else fails)

Systemic Consequences

IBD can lead to systemic illness; that's essentially what this book is all about. It's covered in the rest of the manual, so I don't propose to dwell on it here.

This is just about the local effects of inflammation on the lining and functions of the bowel itself. OK?

However, one common problem I have not mentioned elsewhere is the significant loss of blood from the digestive tract, leading to frank anemia. Anemia means that the amount of healthy red blood cells, which carry oxygen to organs, is below normal. This can make a person feel very tired.

Just note in passing a few other systemic consequences, which can include:

- Arthritis and joint pain

- Weak bones and bone breaks

- Inflammation in the eye and other eye problems

- Liver inflammation

- Gallstones

- Red bumps or ulcers on the skin

- Kidney stones

- Delayed puberty and growth problems (in children and teens)

- In rare cases, lung problems

Some of these problems are caused by malabsorption of nutrients (weak bones and growth problems, for example). Others are due to inflammation in parts of the body other than the digestive tract.

The condition may get better when the IBD is treated. Sometimes separate treatment is needed.

Tests Used To Diagnose IBD

These include:

Blood tests. A sample of blood is studied in a lab to find signs of inflammation and anemia.

Stool sample. A sample of a bowel movement is tested for blood. It is also tested for signs of an infection that can trigger a flare-up of IBD.

Colonoscopy or sigmoidoscopy. For both of these tests, a long, thin tube with a lighted camera inside the tip is inserted into the anus. The image appears on a television screen. A sigmoidocospy allows the doctor to see the lining of the lower part of the large intestine. A colonoscopy goes higher and allows the gastroenterologist to see the lining of the entire large intestine and sometimes even the last part of the small intestines (ouch!)

Any inflammation, bleeding, or ulcers will be seen and it is usal to take a biopsy for the lab.

Barium X-ray. In this classic procedure, a thick, chalky liquid called barium is used to coat the lining of the digestive tract. Then x-rays are taken. Areas coated with barium show up white on x-ray film. This allows the doctor to check for signs of IBD. The barium can be drunk or given as an enema.

Computerized axial tomography (CT or CAT scan). A CT scan takes x-rays from several different angles around the body. The doctor studies the images with a computer to look for signs of ulcerative colitis.

Capsule endoscopy. Regular endoscopies and colonoscopies cannot get to your small intestine. But doctors can examine the small intestine by taking a biopsy sample with a "Crosby capsule". These days it may more sense to pass a tiny, pill shaped camera. You swallow the pill, which then travels through your digestive system. It records video of the small intestine and sends the video to a monitor where your doctor can watch it.

Capsule endoscopies may be dangerous if there is any narrowing of the digestive system and should not be used.

Diet For Irritable Bowel Disease

Numerous studies have shown that avoidance of ALL foods (called total parenteral nutrition or TPN) leads to dramatic improvement in 70 – 90 % of cases of IBD. But such diets are unpalatable, difficult to sustain, expensive, nutritionally incomplete and therefore potentially dangerous.

[Gaby A. "Nutritional Medicine, Fritz Perlberg Publishing, Concord NH, 2011, p. 398]

All the orthodox literature and official sites state plainly that no special eating plan has been proven effective for treating inflammatory bowel disease (IBD). But that's because they don't know my secret: the personal anti-inflammatory foods plan, laid out in my book Diet Wise.

The fact is, if you do it right and eliminate all possible foods that are not tolerated, you can usually get a major recovery. This is really avoiding the foods the microbiota are telling you not to eat; well, do as they say, not as the "experts" say!

Especially avoid advice from licensed dieticians; they are among the most misinformed, as well as the most arrogant, "experts" I know. Their rigid belief in the balanced diet means that they will FORCE you to eat the wrong foods. Their mantra is that if you eat a "balanced diet", the sun will always shine, everyone will be happy, diseases vanish as if by magic and nothing can ever go wrong.

Trouble is, they want you to eat dairy (bad), sugar (very, very bad), grains (even worse) and don't see a problem with manufactured foods (which can be lethal).

Stay away from dieticians; stay alive, that's my dictum.

Advice you will frequently hear from official sources is:

- Avoiding greasy or fried foods

- Avoiding cream sauces and meat products

- Avoiding spicy foods

- Avoiding foods high in fiber, such as nuts and raw fruits and vegetables

- Eating smaller, more frequent meals

- Even though you may have to limit certain foods, you should still aim to eat meals that give you all the nutrients you need.

Better methods of revitalizing the microbiome and reducing inflammation are discussed later in this book. Meantime, here are a couple more details…

The Sulfur Connection

The colon in people with ulcerative colitis tends to contain abnormally high levels of bacteria which breaks down sulfur-containing molecules into hydrogen sulfide and other sulfur metabolites. Sulfur compounds, by the way, are ones that smell strongly and are partly responsible for the offensive odor of pooh.

Sulfur compounds are also poisonous and these metabolites may disrupt the intestinal mucosa, causing actual damage and leakage. They may also suppress butyrates, which feed enterocytes (page 65).

Clinical trials have shown that avoiding sulfur foods; mainly eggs, milk, cheese, garlic and onions, and the cruciferous vegetables (broccoli, cabbage, kale, mustard greens, Brussel sprouts. Etc.) is helpful in ulcerative colitis, simply by lowering sulfur production in the bowel. This seems to be a true effect, independent of any "food allergy" phenomenon.

Test this yourself: break open an uncooked broccoli stem and sniff. It stinks of sulfur!

Gottschalls' Specific Carbohydrate Diet (SCD)

Elaine Gottschall began researching diet, after her four year old daughter developed ulcerative colitis. Her conventional doctor recommended colectomy and became highly abusive when she refused this treatment for her child.

So Gottschall went out on her own. She came across the work of 92- year old Sidney V. Haas, a New York MD, who had spent decades studying the nutritional treatment of colitis. In fact he had what was once a standard nutritional textbook on all medical shelves but then, like so much other good, holistic therapy, it was forgotten about when antibiotics came along. As today, most doctors knew little or nothing about nutrition.

Gottschall's daughter made a full recovery, much to her mothers diet, who ever after became a passionate advocate of the Haas approach.

So really, Haas should get the credit. But I'm afraid that, now, Gottschall's name is going to be forever associated with what has become known as the "specific carbohydrate diet" or SCD. [here let me remind you of the "intestinal carbohydrate fermentation syndrome" I described on page 60. It fits!]

The principle of the plan is avoidance of certain carbohydrates (duh!), for example glucose is OK but fructose is not.

In practice that means:

> No lactose, sucrose, HFCS
>
> No grains (all starchy)
>
> No agar, carrageen or other seaweed derivatives
>
> No starchy legumes
>
> No starchy vegetables (no potato, yams, parsnips, etc.)
>
> No processed meats

You might wonder at the last but in practice processed meat manufacturers often hide sugars in the products, supposedly to make them taste better.

What you can eat safely is the following:

- Unprocessed meats

- Eggs

- Fish

- Most non-starchy vegetables

- Most fruits and juices, especially berries

- Plain yoghurt and lactose-free cheeses

- Nuts, nut flours for baked goods

- Navy, string and lima beans

- Oils, light tea and coffee, distilled alcohols (spirits), honey

My advice is NOT honey. That's naïve. Honey contains a lot of fructose, which is banned.

I think nut milks (unsweetened) would be good though.

You can learn more and practice this approach in detail by getting a copy of Gottschall's book Breaking The Vicious Cycle.

The FODMAP Diet

This is fashionable among conventional doctors at the moment, because it has "science"! It is also about carbohydrates in the diet.

FODMAP stands for fermentable oligo-, di- and monosaccharides and polyols. Foods containing these carbohydrate classes you exclude.

Fruits
Apple, apricot, avocado, blackberries, cherries, lingon, lychee, mango, nashi fruit, nectarine, peach, pear, plum (prune), persimmon, rambutan, watermelon

Grains
Rye, wheat

Legumes
Baked beans, chickpeas, lentils, kidney beans

Vegetables
Artichokes, asparagus, avocado, beets, broccoli, brussel sprouts, cabbage, cauliflower, garlic (with large consumption), fennel, leeks, mushrooms, okra, onions, peas, radiccio, lettuce ,scallions (white parts), shallots, sugar snap peas, snow peas

Try this regime, if you have no luck with anything else. You can get a downloadable, printable chart of FODMAP foods here:

www.fireinthebellybook.com/fodmap-intolerances.pdf

Further IBD Resources

Resources for US patients: (if you want to send me similar resources for other territories, I'll be glad to update the text with them).

More information on inflammatory bowel disease (USA), call womenshealth.gov at 800-994-9662 (TDD: 888-220-5446) or contact the following organizations:

American Gastroenterological Association (http://www.gastro.org)
Phone: 301-654-2055

Crohn's & Colitis Foundation of America, Inc. (http://www.ccfa.org)
Phone: 800-932-2423

National Digestive Diseases Information Clearinghouse, NIDDK, NIH (http://www.digestive.niddk.nih.gov)
Phone: 800-891-5389 (TDD: 866-569-1162)

National Institute of Diabetes & Digestive & Kidney Diseases (http://www2.niddk.nih.gov)
Phone: 301-496-3583

North American Society for Pediatric Gastroenterology, Hepatology and Nutrition (http://www.naspghan.org)
Phone: 215-233-0808

The American College of Gastroenterology (http://gi.org)
Phone: 301-263-9000

Higher Risk Of Getting Cancer

Inflammatory bowel disease (IBD) can increase an individual's chances of getting cancer of the colon. Even so, more than 90 percent of people with IBD do NOT get colon cancer.

Ulcerative colitis is a cancer culprit that goes right back to my med schools days. It was known even then. But current research suggests that Crohn's patients have an increased risk as well. For both diseases, the risk of colon cancer depends on how long the disease has been present. The risk of colon cancer does not start to increase until a patient has had the inflammatory disease for 8 to 10 years, so it's a long-term thing. People whose disease affects the entire colon have the highest risk of colon cancer. People whose disease affects only the rectum have the lowest risk.

Regular colonoscopy is then a must for IBD patients with a disease history of 8 to 10 years or longer.

But now, what about cancer as a systemic disease—cancer in other parts of the body—as a result of "fire in the belly"? This is a good place; let's talk about it here…

Cancer and Inflammation

I have previously hinted at the link between cancers and systemic inflammation. Certain viruses, we know, lead directly to cancer (HPV for one). But it needs stating clearly that cancer is the greatest health hazard we face from any inflammation, specifically including "fire in the belly" and a disordered microbiome.

Recognition of this important connection is currently under much scientific scrutiny but is far from new.

The Roman physician Claudius Galenus observed some similarity between cancer and inflammation almost 2 thousand years ago. Galen originally used Hippocrates's term "cancer" specifically to describe certain inflammatory tumors of the breast in which superficial veins appeared swollen and radiated, somewhat like the claws of a crab. Later the name was extended to include all malignant and infiltrating growths.

In 1863 Rudolf Virchow noted white blood cells or leukocytes in neoplastic tissues and made a connection between inflammation and cancer. He suggested that this immune cell infiltrate reflected the origin of cancer at sites of chronic inflammation.

A seminal observation was made more than a century later, when Harold Dvorak of Harvard University noted that inflammation and cancer share some basic developmental mechanisms (angiogenesis) and tissue-infiltrating cells (lymphocytes, macrophages, and mast cells), and that tumors act like "wounds that do not heal."

This suspicion that inflammation leads to cancer, is indirectly supported by the observation that taking aspirin daily for 5 years or longer can protect against death from colorectal and other solid cancers. In trials in which the patients had been taking aspirin for more than 7.5 years, the 20-year risk of cancer death (from the initiation of the trials) was reduced by approximately 30 percent for all solid cancers and by 60 percent for gastrointestinal cancers. For lung and esophageal cancer, the benefit was confined to subtypes of those cancers that originated in glandular tissue (adenocarcinomas). For colorectal cancer, the effect was high for cancer in the proximal colon but not in the distal colon.

[http://f1000.com/reports/m/3/11] .

I'm not suggesting the use of aspirin, merely to point out that it blocks inflammation and at the same time seems to reduce the incidence of cancer. This is more than a coincidence.

The data clearly points to the fact that significantly reducing inflammation in the body will prevent the initiation and progression of both gastrointestinal and other solid organ cancers (including lung and prostate), and suggest that inflammation may be an underlying cause of cancer even in tumor types that had not been traditionally thought to originate within chronically inflamed tissues.

Bacteria, Inflammation, And Cancer

Gut microbes are increasingly being linked to diverse medical conditions including obesity, inflammatory bowel disease, diabetes, and cancer.

One example of a cancerous gut microbe is Helicobacter pylori—a bacterium that resides in the GI tract of almost two-thirds of the world's population, and is responsible for stomach ulcers in many people.

Gastric mucosa-associated lymphoid tissue (MALT) lymphoma is a cancer that occurs in the stomach and is frequently associated with H. pylori. One benefit, then, of taking antibiotics, is that ridding the patient of this bacterium causes this particular cancer to regress in upwards of 80 percent of these patients, and half are cured.

However, the more usual gastric cancer, is not helped by antibiotics and remains a difficult and very dangerous cancer. Of course, harboring this bacterium does not automatically lead to cancer: the guts of some 4.5 billion people are home to H. pylori, yet stomach cancer occurs in only a fraction of individuals.

Bacteroides fragilis has been shown to initiate colon cancer in mice and may also do so in humans. This bacterium's toxin is a metalloprotease which is best known as a master regulator of inflammatory response pathways. In this and other ways, this bacterial strain drives inflammation, which creates conditions that promote cancer formation and progression. Much of the current thinking about how bacteria may contribute to cancers, particularly those of the gastrointestinal tract, involves chronic inflammation. (See "An Aspirin for your Cancer?" The Scientist, April 2011.)

Finally (these are only examples and there are plenty more), Agrobacterium tumefaciens is a soil phytopathogen that reliably elicits neoplastic growths [ie. cancer] on the host plant species. We just don't know if it has any pathological effect on human cells.

It has been shown to cause genetic changes in the famous HeLa cells, a human cancer line that's been running for over 60 years.

[Genetic Transformation Of Hela Cells By Agrobacterium, Proceedings of the National Academy Sciences USA, 10.1073/pnas.041327598]

Chapter 8 Degenerative Disorder (Autism) and Fire In The Belly

Many of you will know that an English surgeon Andrew Wakefield published a notorious paper in The Lancet in February 1998.

He found abnormal measles virus in the guts of children with autism. The virus was out of place, highly inflammatory and a rogue species, developed for vaccination purposes. You have heard me endlessly, over the years, defend Wakefield and try to talk people out of the mercury-in-vaccines hypothesis as a cause of autism. It isn't.

I know what causes autism and I have been saying so since 1983, when I had my first of a series of cases of severe autistic disorder (at that time called disintegrative psychosis). All of my cases, without exception, started within days of a measles shot. The child got worse and ended up in a disastrous condition. This was clear because it was in the days before MMR (measles combined with mumps and rubella).

The measles vaccine was to blame, I said so, I went on radio with Gay Byrne in Dublin to say so, and I've been saying it ever since.

Andrew Wakefield just put the science behind my considerable clinical experience of this.

Well, all Hell broke loose when Wakefield published. Big Pharma, with their bully-boy pals in the media, set out to utterly discredit him. Boy, they did an evil job.

They sent in an "investigative" reporter, called Brian Deer —not even a scientific enquiry team— to make up lies and trash Wakefield's reputation.

Andrew was accused of having "financial interest" in this study and faking his findings, in the desperate attempt to make everyone think that vaccines are safe and Wakefield is a money hungry liar.

He is supposed to have manufactured a claim that the children he studied suffered from a kind of non-specific colitis (fire in the gut, to us).

In February 2010, The Lancet formally retracted Wakefield's 1998 paper. The retraction states that "the claims in the original paper that children were 'consecutively referred' and that investigations were 'approved' by the local ethics committee have been proven to be false"

[The Editors Of The Lancet (February 2010). "Retraction—Ileal-lymphoid-nodular hyperplasia, non-specific colitis, and pervasive developmental disorder in children". Lancet 375 (9713): 445. doi:10.1016/S0140-6736(10)60175-4. PMID 20137807]

The full implication was that Wakefield was massaging figures for financial gain. The derisory corollary was that The Lancet would never publish such a travesty of science, when in fact they do it all the time, as a favor to their advertisers from Big Pharma. But the damage was done (as intended).

The following day the editor of a specialist journal, Neurotoxicology, withdrew another Wakefield paper that was in press. The article, which concerned research on monkeys, had already been published online and sought to implicate vaccines in autism.

In May 2010, The American Journal of Gastroenterology retracted a paper of Wakefield's that used data from the 12 patients of the Lancet article.

On 5 January 2011, BMJ editors recommended that Wakefield's other publications should be scrutinized and retracted if need be. Effectively, Andrew Wakefield's career was destroyed. A massive blow had been struck for ignorance and stupidity.

Yet what Andrew Wakefield, then a reader in gastroenterology at the Royal Free Hospital in North London, and 12 other doctors found is incontestable: many of the children with autistic disorder had a rogue measles virus in their gut. It was a new kind of bowel disease, autism enterocolitis.

In the rush to destroy his credibility and reputation, nobody actually said he didn't find this connection (did you notice that?)

At the time, Dr Wakefield said that although they had not proved a link between MMR (measles, mumps, rubella) and autism, there was cause for concern and the Government should offer the option single vaccines - instead of only MMRs - until more research had been done.

Wakefield never said stop all vaccines; he merely suggested maybe we could just give all three separately for a time, until this matter could be further researched. He didn't even say the virus he found had caused the autism; only that there was a statistical correlation. Pretty modest, you would say? But it got him assassinated professionally, because it wasn't to the liking of those who want to peddle forced vaccinations on all children.

In February 2002, Wakefield issued a surprising statement, accused the industry of, Treating the public as though they are some kind of moronic mass who cannot make an informed decision for themselves."

[Wakefield, Andrew (2002-02-10). "Why I owe it to parents to question triple vaccine". Sunday Herald. Archived from the original on 2003-08-03. Retrieved 2007-08-10.]

Now new revelations have made it more than clear that the BMJ in January 2011 alleging that Wakefield falsified data, were in fact the real fraudulent claims in this story. The attack on Wakefield was a pack of lies from Brian Deer, for which, one assumes, he duly received his 30 pieces of silver and cares not a whit for the children jeopardized by his money hungry lies.

There continues to be no statement that what he found didn't exist. It's just blurred by the classic tactic of muddying the waters; Wakefield, Deer said, planned to start a company to make money out of his discovery. So what? That's the entire reason for scientific papers published in journals: Big Pharma is doing it because it intends to make money out of the study!!

Consider this shock revelation

Research microbiologist David Lewis, of the National Whistleblowers Center, explains that he reviewed histopathological grading sheets by two of Dr. Wakefield's coauthors, pathologists Amar Dhillon and Andrew Anthony, and concluded there was no fraud committed by Dr. Wakefield:

"As a research microbiologist involved with the collection and examination of colonic biopsy samples, I do not believe that Dr. Wakefield intentionally misinterpreted the grading sheets as evidence of "non-specific colitis." Dhillon indicated "non-specific" in a box associated, in some cases, with other forms of colitis. In addition, if Anthony's grading sheets are similar to ones he completed for the Lancet article, they suggest that he diagnosed "colitis" in a number of the children."

"The grading sheets and other evidence in Wakefield's files clearly show that it is unreasonable to conclude, based on a comparison of the histological records, that Andrew Wakefield 'faked' a link between the MMR vaccine and autism."

Nothing is plainer than that: two independent skilled pathologists (not "investigative journalists") looked at the data and stated clearly there is no evidence of any kind of fraud by Andrew Wakefield.

That's sad. But what is more horrific in a story like this is the millions of children's lives betrayed by deliberate lies, manipulated just to protect profits. It's money before truth. Brain Deer is a socio-path of the highest order.

The real point is that the science here is not about whether Andrew Wakefield is twisted or incompetent. He, isn't. It's about the fact that there appears to be a connection between inflammation, and particularly gut inflammation, and autism. In other words "fire in the belly" connects strongly to the autism story.

See, what you will not have heard or read—because the US media exert terrific censorship on their "free" citizens—is that plenty of other research has since confirmed Wakefield's hotly contested findings.

In 2006 a British newspaper The Daily Mail reported

" … a team from the Wake Forest University School of Medicine in North Carolina are examining 275 children with regressive autism and bowel disease - and of the 82 tested so far, 70 prove positive for the measles virus … the team's leader, Dr Stephen Walker, said: 'Of the handful of results we have in so far, all are vaccine strain and none are wild measles.

'This research proves that in the gastrointestinal tract of a number of children who have been diagnosed with regressive autism, there is evidence of measles virus.

'What it means is that the study done earlier by Dr Wakefield and published in 1998 is correct. That study didn't draw any conclusions about specifically what it means to find measles virus in the gut, but the implication is it may be coming from the MMR vaccine. If that's the case, and this live virus is residing in the gastrointestinal tract of some children, and then they have GI inflammation and other problems, it may be related to the MMR.'

The lead researcher, Stephen J. Walker, Ph.D., was also quick to state however, that this does not necessarily mean the MMR vaccine causes autism. Still, his research notes the same connection that Wakefield's team did, which is that many autistic children have chronic bowel inflammation, and have the vaccine strain of the measles virus in their intestines.

[Sally Beck, Mail on Sunday, 05/28/2006]

Further…

Documents revealed early in 2011 showed that on December 20th, 1996, a meeting of The Inflammatory Bowel Disease Study Group based at the Royal Free Hospital Medical School featured a presentation by Professor Walker-Smith on seven of the children who would later become part of the group of patients Dr Wakefield wrote about in his 1998 The Lancet paper (which was later retracted by The Lancet).

Remember, Dr Wakefield has been accused of completely fabricating his findings about these same children in his 1998 paper, but these documents reveal that fourteen months before Dr Wakefield's paper was published, two other researchers -- Professor Walker-Smith and Dr Amar Dhillon -- independently documented the same problems in these children, including symptoms of autism

Professor Walker-Smith's 1996 presentation at the Royal Free Hospital Medical School was entitled, "Entero-colitis and Disintegrative Disorder Following MMR - A Review of the First Seven Cases."

Prof. Walker-Smith said at that meeting, "I wish today, to present some preliminary details concerning seven children, all boys, who appear to have entero-colitis and disintegrative disorder, probably autism, following MMR."

Says Dr. Wakefield of his original 1998 findings

"… it's been replicated in Canada, in the U.S., in Venezuela, in Italy… [but] they never get mentioned. All you ever hear is that no one else has ever been able to replicate the findings. I'm afraid that is false."

From Joe Mercola's site, I found a list of 28 studies supporting Wakefield's finding (as of April 2010, there are probably over a hundred by now):

1. The Journal of Pediatrics November 1999; 135(5):559-63
2. The Journal of Pediatrics 2000; 138(3): 366-372
3. Journal of Clinical Immunology November 2003; 23(6): 504-517
4. Journal of Neuroimmunology 2005
5. Brain, Behavior and Immunity 1993; 7: 97-103
6. Pediatric Neurology 2003; 28(4): 1-3
7. Neuropsychobiology 2005; 51:77-85
8. The Journal of Pediatrics May 2005;146(5):605-10
9. Autism Insights 2009; 1: 1-11
10. Canadian Journal of Gastroenterology February 2009; 23(2): 95-98
11. Annals of Clinical Psychiatry 2009:21(3): 148-161
12. Journal of Child Neurology June 29, 2009; 000:1-6
13. Journal of Autism and Developmental Disorders March 2009;39(3):405-13
14. Medical Hypotheses August 1998;51:133-144.
15. Journal of Child Neurology July 2000; ;15(7):429-35
16. Lancet. 1972;2:883–884.
17. Journal of Autism and Childhood Schizophrenia January-March 1971;1:48-62
18. Journal of Pediatrics March 2001;138:366-372.
19. Molecular Psychiatry 2002;7:375-382.
20. American Journal of Gastroenterolgy April 2004;598-605.
21. Journal of Clinical Immunology November 2003;23:504-517.
22. Neuroimmunology April 2006;173(1-2):126-34.
23. Prog. Neuropsychopharmacol Biol. Psychiatry December 30 2006;30:1472-1477.
24. Clinical Infectious Diseases September 1 2002;35(Suppl 1):S6-S16
25. Applied and Environmental Microbiology, 2004;70(11):6459-6465
26. Journal of Medical Microbiology October 2005;54:987-991

27. Archivos venezolanos de puericultura y pediatría 2006; Vol 69 (1): 19-25.
28. Gastroenterology. 2005:128 (Suppl 2);Abstract-303

What has slowly emerged, despite every effort to suppress the truth, is that autism and bowel disturbance, typical of "Fire In The belly" seem to go together, exactly as my cases, starting in 1983, seemed to show.

There is also the possibility that the rise in autism we are seeing be due to the fact that mother's are passing on to their children a very disturbed bowel flora. That initial inoculation, as we have seen (page 52), is crucial to teaching not only the immune system but the nervous system too.

Dr. Campbell-McBride discovered that nearly all of the mothers of autistic children have abnormal gut flora. Babies who develop abnormal gut flora are left with compromised immune systems, putting them at higher risk for suffering vaccine reactions.

But they also develop mentally in a different way too. There are detectable physical brain differences.

With this in mind, correcting disordered bowel flora and quenching the "fire in the belly" becomes a quest of extraordinary concern for any woman embarking on pregnancy. This is especially so if the mother has a history of taking antibiotics with any frequency.

What's more every child should be tested for healthy bowel flora before a vaccination is even considered. This ridiculous notion of giving infants, across the board, the same doses of a powerful medication like a vaccine plus its excipients (added extras), is in violation of all medical wisdom.

We are all different, as I explained in the section on DNA variations called SNPs. Some children simply cannot handle the huge burden on their immune system. As a result, they are damaged for life.

But because admitting it would hamper Big Pharma profits, lies are told, good men and women brought down… and, of course, millions of children hurt.

Other Potential Causative Organisms

However, the truth is far from clear. It may not be as simple as one virus. Another gut organism is being looked at too: a bacterium called *Sutterella wadsworthensis*.

According to new research conducted in the Center for Infection and Immunity (CII) at Columbia University's Mailman School of Public Health, children with autism and gastrointestinal disturbances have high levels of Sutterella in their intestines.

In their report, published Jan. 10, 2012, in the online journal mBio, researchers from the Mailman School of Public Health at Columbia University in New York City suggested that this finding could help explain the link between autism and gastrointestinal problems, such as inflammation.

The investigators found that over half of the children diagnosed with autism and gastrointestinal disturbances had Sutterella in intestinal biopsy tissue, while Sutterella was absent in biopsies from typically developing children with gastrointestinal disturbances. Not only was Sutterella present in the intestines of children with autism, but relative to most genera of bacteria, Sutterella was present at remarkably high levels. Sutterella species have been isolated from human infections previous to this study, but it remains unclear whether this bacterium is a human pathogen.

There is more to be done toward understanding the role Sutterella might play in autism, the microbiota, infections, and inflammation.

Meanwhile, the incidence of autism goes on increasing, despite removing mercury from many childhood vaccines. It is very likely that autism is another variant of what I've christened "Fire In The Belly".

Source: PR Newswire November 10, 2011
Source: BMJ November 9, 2011
Source: Nature 2011, 479, 157-158

You should also read Wakefield's book *Callous Disregard*.

part 2

Quenching The Flames

How To Deal With Fire In The Belly

Quenching Inflammation, then, we have seen is not only desirable but essential to continued good health, slower aging and avoiding the cancer malady.

You need to knockout the likely causes, one by one. You can do more than one action at once but don't take on too much; it will get confusing. The first place to start (always) is removing offending foods, be they food allergies or genetically incompatible foods.

Chapter 9 Is It A Food Allergy Or Intolerance?

I almost invariably recommend a patient with a high score from the inventory of symptoms on page 3, start by trying to identify food allergies and intolerances.

This is not to say that everything is a food allergy. But diet adjustments are a great place to start because there is usually some kind of beneficial result and they are relatively easy to do. If you can feel much better just avoiding, say, milk or wheat, that is far easier than battling against multiple environmental shocks and stressors. The reason is simple if you understand the overload principle: avoiding one stressor, especially if it is an important one, may free your body defenses up enough so that it can cope with the rest, without your help!

Symptoms suggesting food allergy

Bloating and flatulence

Food binges

Food cravings

Overweight, underweight or wildly fluctuating weight (gain a few pounds in a day)

Symptoms actually come on while eating

Symptoms after food (falling asleep, chills, sudden rapid heartbeat)

Feeling unwell when going long periods without food (food addiction)

Feeling tired, crabby or unwell on waking (also a sign of food addiction)

The last may seem strange: most everybody wakes up feeling bad don't they? True, but as I have been teaching for decades, that's because almost everyone is suffering the addiction effects of allergy.

Think about this: by the time we wake in the morning, we may not have eaten for 10- 14 hours; that's more than enough time to set up withdrawal symptoms. With breakfast, we get our first "fix" of wheat, sugar, caffeine, or whatever and the symptoms start to clear right away. You don't believe me? Wait until you have followed the instruction in this section and you'll see the amazing truth of what I say.

For more in this phenomenon and extra detail and help on exploring the subject of allergy and intolerance foods, you can't do better than get yourself a copy of my best-selling Diet Wise. It will more than repay the study. You can get a copy at: www.DietWiseBook.com

Meantime, this chapter will give you a basic program to work with.

The Secret Of Food Allergy Test Dieting

The secret of successful identification of food allergies is to give up sufficient foods to be able to feel well, then to re-introduce these foods one at a time, so that detecting a reaction is relatively easy. We call this elimination and challenge dieting. It rarely works to give up just one food at a time because anyone who is ill is almost certain to have more than one allergy. If it was simply one major allergen, the person would have spotted it eventually, as indeed some lucky people do.

Dr Doris Rapp of New York coined an instructive term: the "eight nails in the shoe trap". She points out that if you have eight nails sticking out in your shoe, and then pull just one of these nails, you will still not be comfortable – because of the other seven. It can be the same with multiple allergies. You have to work at it just that little bit harder.

Make no mistake, elimination diets can be tough; they should be. But it is important to remember that I am talking here of a trial diet—an experimental procedure you would carry out for a couple of weeks or so. You do not need to stay on a tough diet long-term; indeed you are specifically cautioned not to do so, otherwise you run into problems caused by inadequate nutritional sources.

The purpose of the strict "test" diet is to isolate the culprits. Once you know these, you can eat most anything else. This means you shift into a maintenance diet, solely avoiding these offending foods, something you stay on for months or years. Almost anyone who feels much better by avoiding one or two foods has the will power to continue; the rewards are high!

Please don't mix up these two grades of diet. You'll suffer needlessly.

Three-Tiered Inflammatory Food Elimination and Identification

The rest of this section is given over to discussing three-tiered dieting, from which you can choose the most appropriate approach for you or your family. In following the instructions it is vital that in all cases you also avoid manufactured foods. This is not because food additives are a common intolerance problem (they are surprisingly uncommon, in fact) but because manufactured foods contain numerous foodstuffs that are hidden and disguised, such as corn starch, wheat, sugar, egg and other notable allergens.

Don't trust the labeling, it may be misleading and throw the whole test. Just eat only fresh whole versions of the foods allowed, in other words nothing from tins, packets, bottles and jars. Don't even trust to foods cooked and packages by supermarkets and stores.

It may cost you the results you are looking for.

Special note: people often ask me about using organic foods in an elimination diet. The answer is Yes, it is always better to eat organic, if you can. But that may not be easy and it is not really necessary. Almost everyone will feel better by eating ordinary commercial food supplies, providing they are fresh. Only if you are very sensitive or very poorly, is it recommended that you go the whole nine yards and eat fully organic foods.

A word about drugs

Drug allergies are not rare and it may be wise to discontinue medications which are unnecessary. However, certain drugs are essential and should not be stopped, such as anti-epileptics, some cardiac drugs (such as digoxin), insulin and thyroxin. Some medications, such as cortisone derivatives, need to be phased out gradually.

To be certain, it is better to discuss the implications with your doctor and ask his or her advice on stopping your treatment. Don't be put off by the high-handedness which some doctors, sadly, are prone to when their prescriptions are questioned. You are entitled to know the effect of any drug you are taking and also precisely why you are taking it, and it may be that your doctor will not even understand the workings and side-effects of drugs being used.

The key question that you want answered is, 'Will I come to harm if I stop this drug?' Nine times out of ten the answer is, 'No'.

Don't forget, tobacco is a drug. You must stop smoking if you are serious about getting well.

Now, let's start with the easiest level diet as an entry.

An Easy Elimination Diet (14-21 Days)

It is logical to start by eliminating only the common likely food allergies. This leaves plenty of foods to eat and you should not find this diet too onerous. It is especially suitable for a child and consists basically of fresh meat, fish, fruit and vegetables, with juice and water to drink. We call it the 'Stone-Age' or 'Caveman' diet. (my first nickname with the UK press was "The Stone Age Doctor"; I used to joke this was an unfair exaggeration, I had only a few grey hairs at the time!).

Foods you are allowed to eat:

> Any meat (not processed or smoked)
>
> Any vegetables (fresh or frozen, not tinned)
>
> Any fruit, except the citrus family (lemon etc.)
>
> Any fish (not processed or smoked)
>
> Quinoa (grain substitute)
>
> All fresh unsweetened fruit juices, except citrus
>
> Herb teas (careful: some contain citrus peel)
>
> Spring water, preferably bottled in glass
>
> Fresh whole herbs
>
> Salt and pepper to taste

OK, that's straightforward. There is plenty to eat, in other words. You may have to change what you usually do but you will not starve, that's for sure.

Foods you are not allowed to eat:

- No stimulant drinks – no tea, coffee, alcohol

- No sugar, honey, additives or sweeteners

- No grains: absolutely no wheat, corn, rye, rice, barley, oats or millet. That means no bread, cakes, muffins, biscuits, granola, pastry, flour or farina

- No milk or dairy produce: no skimmed milk, cream, butter, margarines or spreads, not even goat's milk

- NO MANUFACTURED FOOD: nothing from tins, packets, bottles or jars. If somebody labeled it, they likely added to it.

Aspects Of Elimination Dieting

Here are some important points to keep in mind:

It is vital to understand that you must not cheat on this or any other exclusion diet. This is not a slimming diet, where you can sneak a piece of chocolate cake and still lose weight. Remember that it takes several days for food to clear your bowel and eating it as little as twice a week will prevent you clearing it from your system. If you do slip up, you will need to extend the avoidance period for several more days. Later on, when the detective work is complete, the occasional indiscretion won't matter In the meantime, follow the instructions exactly.

Don't forget about addictions. It is quite likely that you will get withdrawal symptoms during the first few days. This is good news because it means you have given up something important. Usually the effects are mild and amount to nothing more than feeling irritable, tired, or perhaps having a headache, but be warned -it could put you in bed for a couple of days. I have seen a wheat exclusion "cold turkey" that was just as grim as narcotics.

Please also note that it is possible to be allergic even to the allowed foods - they are chosen simply because reaction to them is less common. If you are in this minority, you might even feel worse on this diet, but at least it proves you have a food allergy. In that case, try eliminating, also, the foods you are eating more of (potato is a common offender) and see if you then begin to improve. If not, you should switch to the Eight Foods Diet, or a fast as described below.

While on the elimination diet, try to avoid hanging on to a few favourite foods and eating only those. You must eat with variety; otherwise you will risk creating reactions to the foods you are eating repeatedly. It is senseless to go on with old habits. The whole point of exclusion dieting is to make you change what you are doing - it could be making you ill.

Don't worry about special recipes or substitutes at this stage. By the time you have fried, baked, steamed and grilled everything once, the two weeks will almost have passed! If in the long term it transpires that you need to keep off a food, then you can begin searching for an alternative.

Patients usually ask: What about my vitamin and mineral supplements while on an elimination diet, do I need to take those?

While on the elimination diet, try to avoid hanging on to a few favourite foods and eating only those.

The answer is No. Most vitamin and mineral tablets contain hidden food ingredients, such as corn starch. Even those that say "allergy-free" formulas are misleading. They may not be made up with common allergens, such as wheat, corn or soya derivatives; but nevertheless, vegetable ingredients are present, such as rice polishings and potato starch. To call these allergy "safe", or even hypoallergenic, is in my view dishonest.

Don't take the risk, you won't come to any harm without supplements for a short period. This leads on to another major Scott-Mumby Rule:

The biggest and commonest health hazard by far today is not what you are lacking that you should be having, but what you are already taking that you shouldn't! In other words, giving up allergens, toxic or overload items have far more dramatic results in terms of health recovery than supplementing stuff you are deficient in.

How Did You Get On With This Diet?

If you felt a whole lot better, skip to the section on food challenge testing:

Do not, simply because you do not improve or feel any different, make the erroneous assumption that you could not then be allergic to milk, wheat or other banned foods. Remember the eight nails in the shoe? This would be a serious mistake which could bar your road to recovery. You might like to try an alternative exclusion diet. Several are suggested here.

You can, in any case, carry out useful challenge tests, taking a careful note of what happens when you re-introduce a food. Careful! You do not want to hammer a pointed nail back in that shoe!

The Eight Foods Diet (7-14 days)

Not as severe as a fast but tougher than the previous regime, is what can be called the Few Foods Diet; I prefer to use an 8-food plan. Obviously it is more likely to succeed than the previous plan, since you are giving up more foods. Any determined adult could cope with it, but on no account should you subject a child to this diet without his, or her, full and voluntary cooperation. It could produce a severe emotional trauma otherwise (factually, there is rarely a problem -- most children don't want to be ill and will assist you, providing they understand what you are trying to do).

The basic idea is to produce one or two relatively safe foods for each different category we eat. Everyday foods are avoided since these include the common allergens. Thus we would choose fruits such as mango and papaya, not apple and banana; flesh such as duck and rabbit, not beef and pork; quail and ostrich, not chicken. The diet below contains my suggestions. You can vary it somewhat according to what is available to you locally.

A Suggested 8-Foods Diet

Meat, protein	rabbit, venison
Fowl	ostrich or quail
Fruit	mango, kiwi fruit
Vegetables	spinach, turnip
Starch	buckwheat, quinoa

In addition to the stipulated foods, you are allowed salt to taste but not pepper, spring water but not herb teas or juices. Even herbs and pepper must be challenged correctly on introduction. Note that neither of the starch foods are in the grains family.

You can find out what food families are in the appendix.

Potential Problems

The main problem with such a restricted plan is boredom. However there is enough variety here for adequate nourishment over the suggested period of seven to ten days, providing you eat a balance of all eight foods. Exotic fruits can be expensive, but you won't need to eat them for long and, in any case, few people would deny that feeling well is worth any expense.

The chances are that, on a diet like this, you will feel well within a week, but for some conditions, such as eczema and arthritis, you will need to allow a little longer. Be prepared to go the full ten days before deciding that it isn't working.

A variation of this diet is the exotic food diet. Don't worry how many foods you can round up to eat, choose as many as you can find; just make sure they are all unusual, you personally have never eaten them and they are not related to any common food category. You will need to learn about food families (groups of foodstuffs that are related).

The Fast (5-7 days)

Although a fast is the ultimate approach in tracking down hidden food allergies, I don't recommend it lightly. It is quick (fast!), inexpensive and an absolute yes-no statement on whether your illness really is caused by food allergy. Although it can be tough at first, by the morning of the fifth day, you can expect to feel wonderful! That's why fasting is popular as a religious exercise and why sometimes people with a severe attack of gastro-enteritis, who expel almost all the food content of the bowel by diarrhea and vomiting, are suddenly "cured" of some other health condition.

The real problem is that sometimes it can then be difficult to get back on to any safe foods. Everything is unmasked at once and the patient seems to react to everything he or she tries to eat. This can cause great distress.

Undertake a fast only if you are very determined or you still suspect food allergy and the other two approaches have failed.

Fasting is emphatically not suitable for certain categories of patient:
>   Pregnant women
>   Children
>   Diabetics
>   Epileptics
>   Anyone seriously weakened or debilitated by chronic illness
>   Anyone who has been subject to severe emotional disturbance (especially those prone to violent outbursts, or those who have tried to commit suicide)

The fast itself is simple enough - just don't eat for four or five days. You must stop smoking. Drink only bottled spring water. The whole point is to empty your bowels entirely of foodstuffs. Thus, if you have any tendency to constipation, take Epsom salts to begin with. If in doubt try an enema! Otherwise the effort may be wasted.

It may help to do what I call a grape-day step-down. This means eating grapes only for a day, as an easy-in step towards fasting.

Special note: A variation, which I call the 'half fast', is to eat only two foods, such as lamb and pears. This means taking a gamble that neither lamb nor pears are allergenic, and it is not as sure-fire as the fast proper. It is permissible to carry this out for seven days, but on no account go on for longer than this.

Food Challenge Testing

Whichever elimination approach you use, you will want to move on to testing foods, to see which are inflammatory in nature.

As soon as you feel well on an elimination regime, you can begin testing, although you must not do so before the four day unmasking period has elapsed. Allow longer if you have been constipated.

Of course, you may never improve on an elimination diet. The problem may be something else, not a food. In that case, when three weeks (maximum) have elapsed on the simple elimination diet, two weeks on the Eight Foods Diet, or seven days on a fast, then you must begin re-introducing foods. This is vital. It is not enough to feel well on a very restricted diet; we want to know why? What are the culprits? These are the foods you must avoid long-term, not all those which are banned at the beginning.

Even if you don't feel well, as already pointed out, this does not prove you have no allergies amongst the foods you gave up. Test the foods as you re-introduce them, anyway - you may be in for a surprise.

My recommended procedure is as follows, except for those coming off a fast:

1. Eat a substantial helping of the food, preferably on its own for the first exposure. Lunch is the ideal meal for this.
2. Choose only whole, single foods, not mixtures and recipes. Try to get supplies that have not been chemically treated in any way.
3. Wait several hours to see if there is an immediate reaction, and if not, eat some more of it, along with a typical ordinary evening meal.
4. You may eat a third, or fourth, portion if you want, to be sure.
5. Take your resting pulse (sit still for two minutes) before, and several times during the first 90 minutes after the first exposure to the food. A rise of ten or more beats in the resting pulse is a fairly reliable sign of an allergy. However no change in the pulse does not mean the food is safe, unless symptoms are absent also.

Alkali Salts

If you do experience an unpleasant reaction, take Epsom salts. That will clear the food rapidly form your bowel.

Also, take alkali salts (a mixture of two parts sodium bicarbonate to one part potassium bicarbonate: one teaspoonful in a few ounces of lukewarm water) should help. You can buy alkali salts on the Internet.

Discontinue further tests until symptoms have abated once more. This is very important, as you cannot properly test when symptoms are already present; you are looking for foods which trigger symptoms.

Using the above approach, you should be able to reliably test one food a day, minimum. Go rapidly if all is well, because the longer you stay off a food, the more the allergy (if there is one) will tend to die down and you may miss it.

Occasionally, patients experience a 'build up' which causes confusion and sometimes failure. Suspect this if you felt better on an exclusion diet, but you gradually became ill again when re-introducing foods, and can't really say why. Perhaps there were no noticeable reactions.

In that case, eliminate all the foods you have re-introduced until your symptoms clear again, and then re-introduce them more slowly. This time, eat the foods steadily, several times a day for three to four days before making up your mind. It is unlikely that one will slip the net with this approach.

Once you have accepted a food as safe, of course you must then stop eating it so frequently; otherwise it may become an allergy. Eat it once a day at most - only every four days when you have enough 'safe' foods to accomplish this.

Special Instructions For Those Coming Off A Fast

Ending a fast, we do things differently. You go faster but you must take care and DO NOT start with the obvious, tempting foods, like bread, coffee etc.

Begin only with exotic foods which you don't normally eat! The last thing you want to happen is to get a reaction when beginning to re-introduce foods – it will mean you cannot carry on adding foods until the symptoms settle down once again.

Instead, for the first few days, you want to build up a minimum range of 'safe' foods that you can fall back on. Papaya, rabbit, artichoke and dogfish are the kind of thing to aim for - do the best you can with what is available according to your resources.

The other important point is that you cannot afford the luxury of bringing in one new food a day: you need to go faster than this. When avoided even for as little as two weeks, a cyclical food allergy can die down and you may miss the proof of allergy you are looking for. It is possible to test two or even three foods a day when coming off a fast. Pay particular attention to the pulse rate before and after each test meal and keep notes. It is important to grasp that some symptom, even if not very striking, usually occurs within the first 60 minutes when coming off a fast. You need to be alert to this, or you will miss items and fail to improve without understanding why.

If the worst happens and you are ill by the end of the day and can't say why, condemn all that day's new foods.

The buildup of foods is cumulative: that is, you start with Food A. If it is OK then the next meal is Food A + Food B, then A + B + C and so on.

An example table of foods tests might be:

Days 1- 4
no food

Day 5
breakfast - poached salmon

lunch - mango (plus salmon)

dinner - steamed spinach (plus salmon and mango)

Day 6
breakfast - baked pheasant, quail or partridge + day 5

lunch - kiwi fruit + day 5

dinner - steamed marrow or zucchini (courgette) + day 5

Day 7
breakfast -lamb chop (plus any of the above) + days 5,6

lunch - baked potato (do not eat the skin) + days 5,6

dinner - banana + days 5,6 etc...

Grapes not allowed on day 5, if you used a grape-day step-down

All safe foods are kept up after an allergic reaction. Therefore, if Food F causes a reaction, while you are waiting for it to clear up, you can go on eating foods A-E, until symptoms clear.

Within a few days, you should have plenty to eat, albeit monotonous. From then on, you can proceed as for those on elimination diets if you wish.

Your Personal Exclusion Program

Whichever program you chose, once you have carried out the challenge tests you will have a list of items which you are intolerant of. You must now avoid these, if you are serious about your health. You have, in effect, designed your own personal diet plan for health. Use it as something you return to in times of trouble or stress, a safe platform.

There should be no rush to try and re-introduce any of these items, if at all. Design your living and eating plan without them, long-term. However the good news is that allergies do settle down, sometimes quite rapidly, especially if you pay attention to everything else I have explained in this book. If you develop and practice a newer safer ecological lifestyle, you may have surprisingly little further trouble.

You may feel better than you have felt in years. Many patients feel and act younger, so much so that friends and relatives often comment. I noticed this over thirty years ago and that is one of the reasons I now find myself part of the anti-aging movement.

Another Scott-Mumby maxim: a low allergy diet is the finest possible cosmetic agent for a woman's skin! She glows!

If you find your personal diet plan oppressive because you discovered quite a few reacting foods, then consider desensitization. This is covered in my book Diet Wise.

Food Diary

It is a good idea to keep a food diary during your experiments with food. Write down everything you eat at each meal, or between meals, and also mark in any symptoms which you experience, with the time of onset in relation to meals. It is often possible to spot a pattern which recurs time and time again but which is not evident when relying only on short-term memory.

Warning: a food diary does tend to make you very conscious of food, which is probably a good thing in the short term. However, taking the long view, try to avoid the exercise making you too introverted about feelings and symptoms, otherwise it can start becoming an obsession. Many allergy patients become so consumed by anxiety about what they are eating that they cannot eat or socialize normally. Food allergy investigations, as described here, are merely a tool not an end and should not become a way of life, otherwise family and friends will feel excluded and that in turn leads to rejection.

Many "amateur" gung-ho food allergy books actually tend to create this major social incompetence, because the authors do not have sufficient experience to be aware of the dangers (and likely because they too are obsessive). Make no mistake, food allergy restrictions can ruin relationships and break up marriages, if it is taken to extreme, as many know to their cost. I do not automatically take the patient's side but sympathize with both points of view (because ultimately I see this as in the patient's broader interests).

Eating can become a psychological burden on the patient and intolerable nuisance to family and friends, if you go too far. True health does not mean isolation from society, it means full social wellbeing included in the deal.

The food diary is merely a tool and should be discontinued as soon as practicable.

Alternative Allergy Exclusion Diets

If the simple exclusion diet has not worked, you might like to consider alternative eliminations.

For example, you could try following a meat-free diet. Some people do feel better as vegetarians, certainly: but probably more feel ill because of the high incidence of grain and dairy allergies, as grains and dairy products are staple foods for vegetarians.

Organic Food

Some people (only a few) are better avoiding food treated with chemicals. A diet avoiding this sort of commercial produce is called 'organic'. It is easier nowadays to follow such an eating regime than formerly. Try it if you have reason to suspect you may be reacting to chemicals but don't go overboard: many people are convinced that pesticides on food make them ill but fail to detect them when challenged double-blind.

Organic food suppliers belong to various bodies to help promote themselves and their ideas. Try to make contact with these organizations and find out about your local suppliers. The Henry Doubleday Research organization is a good place to start (see the Useful Addresses section). They have been pioneers in organic farming methods for decades. They can usually supply a list of vendors. The Soil Association even goes so far as to vet produce showing the label 'organic'. Look for their sign of approval but be warned: this is not a legal requirement and anyone can call their wares 'organic' whether they have used chemicals or not.

Your local health food shop should also be able to help find locally-grown supplies.

Gluten-Free

Probably the oldest established allergy to food is hypersensitivity to gluten. It is a sticky protein that is found in wheat, rye, oats and barley and gives rise to the special gluey cooking texture these foods have.

The result of a gluten allergy used to be a very serious wasting condition known as celiac disease or sprue; the patient simply starved with malnutrition, despite eating adequately. It was eventually discovered that gluten allergy was damaging the lining of the intestine so that it couldn't perform properly. This meant that food was not being digested and absorbed properly.

Another condition known to have a definite connection width gluten sensitivity is dermatitis herpetiformis. This is a blistering, intensely itchy rash that usually affects the outer surface of the elbows, buttocks and knees but can occur on any part of the body.

Personally, I think that a lot of the people who get well on a gluten-free diet do so because they are wheat allergic. They can tolerate rye, oats or barley with impunity, so gluten cannot be the offender.

Try a gluten-free diet if you are suspicious, but you must be prepared to stick at it for a minimum of six to eight weeks to be sure of feeling any benefit.

The GFMF Diet

There is a big fad for the GFMF (gluten-free, milk-free) diet at present. This sort of obsession misses the crucial point: that all food reactions are different. People vary a lot and to imagine this simplistic elimination even approximately covers needs is very naïve.

Absolutely any foodstuff can cause reactions. I have seen carrots, lettuce and even spring water cause severe inflammatory reactions.

True, many people will dramatically improve on eliminating just these two foods. But many won't and then may draw the erroneous conclusion they don't have food allergies.

Don't fall for it.

Special Dieting Cases

For most people the problems of exclusion diets are few. Withdrawal symptoms, extra expense or the sloth encountered in changing the habits of a lifetime are the main difficulties. However, two situations require extra comment:

Children

Children have more food allergy problems than adults. Yet food is vital to them; their growth will be stunted if nutrition is inadequate. Consider the size of a newborn infant in relation to that of an adult and you will see at once the wisdom in the old adage 'You are what you eat'.

Whatever dietary experiments are under-taken with children it is vital therefore to see they get adequate substitutes. Milk is a problem food. It is by far the most common allergen in children. The important ingredient in milk, I believe, is not really calcium but vitamin D. Fish oils are a good alternative source. Iodine is also vital to prevent stunting and poor mental development. Since most of our supply comes from milk, alternative provision needs to be made for this element also. Kelp or iodized salt should suffice.

If you are faced with complex or long-term eliminations for your child it is important to weigh him or her regularly (at least once a week) and keep a record of growth. Body size can be compared with charts showing average ranges for males and female youngsters and also percentiles for those who are clearly above or below average, showing how fast they too should be gaining weight. If weight gain is affected you must get help or discontinue what you are doing. Almost no condition (the possible exception being retarded mental growth occurring because of a food allergy) is worth stunting your child's growth. It is better to defer treatment until the child is older.

Remember that withdrawal symptoms can be experienced by children, too. Be very tolerant for the first few days. He or she may crave favorite foods: just say 'No' firmly and offer an alternative. Eventually, hunger will be on your side.

It's remarkable to watch how a youngster who is a faddy eater (a reliable sign of food allergy) suddenly finds his or her appetite and begins to eat heartily.

Children have more food allergy problems than adults.

126

Diabetics

For diabetic patients managed by drugs and diet alone, there should be little problem with an elimination diet. Those on insulin, however, must be very careful about embarking on a low-carbohydrate diet and should not do so without medical supervision.

The simplest modification of the basic exclusion diet is to eat rice as a source of carbohydrate. Quinoa is a good food that fits this context also, if you can obtain it. Better still is to cut down your insulin gradually and reduce your starch intake similarly – under the supervision of your doctor.

The best challenge test to perform (if you have a glucometer and can use it) is to monitor which foods increase your blood glucose. If you haven't a glucometer, just carry out the challenge tests in the normal way.

Psychiatric Patients

Some care needs to be taken when the patient has pronounced mental problems, that is to say severe enough to have been admitted to a psychiatric ward or hospital. Psychiatrists and psychologists have a pronounced blind spot when it comes to physical causes of mental illness. Many reject this possibility outright, yet doctors who practice my kind of medicine have seen many people helped by a simple change of diet and lifestyle.

Food reactions can be so severe as to precipitate mania and psychotic delusion; this sometimes has to be seen to be believed. The common diagnosis "depression" very often means that the patient feels miserable, due to their hidden allergy, and no-one has solved the problem. That is enough to make anyone feel depressed.

This all means that it is not only permissible but desirable to investigate any psychiatric state in this way. But caution is required: I have already referred in this book to a young Irish patient who went on a murderous rampage when he ate certain foods. I am pleased to say that the law courts were willing to accept my evidence that this was not only possible but demonstrated it for the entire nation on prime-time TV. Obviously if this individual had been put on an elimination diet and then challenged with the danger foods, without skilled supervision, someone could have been hurt very badly or even paid with their lives.

Equally serious, is the possibility that the patient may try to injure him or herself, or even try to commit suicide, when challenged in this way.

To learn more about the influence of food and other allergens on state of mind, read my book Diet Wise. You can get a copy at: www.DietWiseBook.com

Chapter 10 **Nutrition Against Inflammation**

OK, we've figured out what you shouldn't eat; now let's look at what you should eat . That means avoiding all identified inflammatory foods, of course, and this is where my system differs greatly from those with less skill and experience.

Even if a food is supposed to be good for you, if it's on your no-no list, you must avoid it. "Experts" who list all the foods that are "good for you", without mentioning the phenomenon of food allergy and intolerance are being silly. I already mentioned a boy who was allergic to any foods in the carrot family—it caused him to have epileptic fits—well what if some smart alec nutritionist

said he must drink carrot juice, it's a powerful nutritional, and that vegetables, including celery and parsnip are good to eat?

You can see what I mean. So when I give you classes of foods that are anti-inflammatory in principle, the previous chapter comes first and takes priority (I put it before this one for a very good reason).

Antioxidants

It's important to understand that free radicals produce inflammatory-type damage. That's the main way in which they harm us. So antioxidants can be predicted to have a powerful inflammatory effect—and they do.

Quenching free radicals quenches inflammation just as surely. That's why this class of foods is very important to us.

Oxygen is essential for the basic functioning of all life-forms. Without it we would die in a matter of minutes. However, it has long been known that oxygen is toxic to cells. Hydrogen peroxide, which vigorously gives off 'live' oxygen, is used as an antiseptic to kill microbes. This 'excited' oxygen strips off the lipid (fatty) envelope surrounding the cell walls, making them collapse. It is equally inimical to bacteria, viruses and yeasts.

In fact white blood cells in our immune system have a peroxidation mechanism for producing this 'live' oxygen on the spot, precisely for the purpose of attacking foreign organisms. Fortunately Nature also sees fit to supply an enzyme – peroxidase – to get rid of it as fast as it is formed; otherwise it would harm the body's own cells.

Even so, this highly active oxygen produced in the tissues is likely to react with other molecules nearby, energizing them and making them in turn super-reactive and hungry to grab onto something – any nearby atoms become 'free radicals'. They too can damage the body inappropriately and we now believe that certain degenerative diseases such as other arthritis conditions, loss of immunity and allergies, cancer and possibly the process of ageing itself are all in some way bound up with this unwanted oxidation process.

However, the mere existence of these radicals does not pose a threat. It wouldn't make sense for Nature to ensure harm. Instead, it seems the damaging effect of oxidation is only made manifest by existing weaknesses in the tissues. We know that nutritional deficits, for example, can make normal healthy cells vulnerable. Lack of selenium, copper, manganese and zinc can each result in increased susceptibility to free-radical damage of the fat part of cell membranes.

Nutrients that we now believe are provided by Nature as a means of combating free radicals we call anti-oxidants. These include beta-carotene, vitamin A, vitamin E, vitamin C, Selenium-containing amino acids (such as cystine) and enzymes such as glutathione reductase, peroxidase (catalase) and superoxide dismutase.

Trace elements are vital for integrity of this anti-oxidant system of enzyme defenses. Thus, for example, glutathione and super-oxide dismutase require copper, manganese and zinc. However, excessive copper (or iron) can actually increase free-radical production.

> Nutrients that we now believe are provided by Nature as a means of combating free radicals we call anti-oxidants.

Extraneous Factors

Foods, as we have seen, can be major exciters of inflammation. But our environment also subjects us to what we term 'oxidative stress': atmospheric pollution, especially petrochemical smog, produces potent oxidants such as ozone, nitrogen dioxide, peroxyacetyl nitrates and other hydrocarbon-derived free radical substances are powerful inflammation exciters.

Here we get a crossover with "fire in the belly". Many chemical pollutants which enter our bodies are now known to reside in belly fat. There is something different about belly fat from most other fatty tissue in our bodies, making it susceptible to deposits of pesticides, halogenated hydrocarbons, PCBs and other deadly toxins.

Don't forget ionizing radiation (radioactivity), which is damaging precisely because it produces free radicals by destabilizing existing molecules (ions are free radicals). We are all subject to a certain degree of 'natural' radiation of this sort, with or without additional man-made sources. With man-made events like Chernobyl and Fukushima, we are also drenched in extra free radicals, with resultant excitation of inflammation.

We eat and breathe radio-activity, so it too is part of the "fire belly" response.

Smoking (active and passive) subjects the lungs and other organs to chronic oxidative stress. Xenobiotic chemicals – including medical and street drugs – can also be sources of oxidative stress.

Poisons can do it, a rather special but still significant version of "fire in the belly." The toxicity of the pesticide parquat, for example, is believed to result from its free radical form. It is made a free radical by the action of an enzyme on the paraquat molecule in the presence of NADPH (nicotinamide dinucleotide phosphate with an added hydrogen atom, a detoxifying co-enzyme). The transformation results in the removal of one electron (reduction).

In the presence of oxygen this paraquat free radical generates a superoxide radical, which attacks lipid membranes. This step takes away the excess electron, returning the paraquat to its original form, ready to start all over again. This can go on indefinitely, each time using up the body's precious stores of co-enzymes. It means that paraquat cannot be adequately metabolized and removed from the body. The victim dies slowly and painfully.

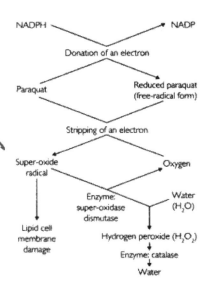

These reactions are probably easier to see diagrammatically and are shown in the figure to the right. It will also show you how oxidative molecules are produced in the tissues (the super-oxide radical on the left, created by stripping electrons from tissue substances) and these markedly damage cell membranes.

Metabolism of a paraquat molecule

130

Tests

Oxidation stress can be measured by looking at the degree to which the patient's red and white blood cells break up when subjected to a particular dilution of hydrogen peroxide. The more they break up, the less anti-oxidant potential of the individual.

Enzymes such as red cell glutathione peroxidase can also be measured, and if levels are low we know that oxidative stress is high. It makes sense also to measure selenium, manganese, copper, and zinc levels, as well as those of vitamin C, vitamin A, vitamin E, and beta-carotene, to get a complete picture of the patient's anti-oxidant status before embarking on treatment.

What To Do

The reader will see that increasing anti-oxidant potential is vital in an increasingly xenobiotic world. Fortunately, this isn't difficult to do. Ensuring that you eat a healthy diet is part of it and also making sure that you have adequate supplements of selenium, vitamins E, A and C and beta-carotene.

Be sure to take good quality iodine and "clean" strontium, when radio-activity is in the air.

Note: the recommendations of this section are in direct conflict to the claims of the **Peroxidation (84)** lobby. I do not recommend the peroxide approach, but at least one clinical ecology doctor in the UK uses it extensively.

Lose Weight

You will rapidly see from what I have been saying that weight loss (shedding the toxic fat) is an important part of an anti-inflammatory program. This was reinforced by a study I found on the results of gastric by-pass surgery (fast-action weight loss).

The 2011 study included 15 people who had gastric bypass surgery at Wake Forest University. Six months after surgery, the participants showed a decrease in proteins that cause inflammation associated with type 2 diabetes and cardiovascular disease, and an increase in proteins that reduce such inflammation.

[Surgery for Obesity and Related Diseases, Volume 7, Issue 5 , Pages 618-624, September 2011]

Gary D. Miller, an associate professor at Wake Forest University, said in a university news release, "We're amassing evidence that weight loss is a very important part of changing the way the body's systems work in people with high-risk diseases like diabetes and heart disease."

A previous study by Miller and colleagues found that gastric bypass surgery followed by a healthy diet and exercise reduces abdominal fat known to increase the risk of cancer and other diseases. So this is a serious issue from "fire in the belly".

Is It Important?

You bet. As we get older, we accumulate more and more toxins. In fact, scientists discovered over 63 different chemicals in the bodies of the oldest generation, including PCBs, organochlorine pesticides, brominated flame retardants, perfluorinated chemicals, and more.

A comprehensive survey by the U.S. Centers for Disease Control found 148 different chemicals in the blood and urine samples of 2,400 Americans. More than a quarter of all the samples contained significant amounts of benzo-a-pryene, an important carcinogen and highly inflammatory.

National Geographic Magazine paid nearly $15,000 to test one of their reporters for the presence of 320 different chemicals as part of an undercover investigation into environmental toxins. The level of one chemical used to make flame retardants was so high it would have been considered alarming, even if the reporter had worked in a plant that manufactured the chemical!

A Mount Sinai School of Medicine study found a total of 167 different chemicals in the blood and urine samples of volunteers — an average of 91 toxins each. The toxins included lead, dioxins, PCBs, phthalate DEHP, as well as compounds that have been banned for more than a quarter century.

When your body is unable to breakdown and eliminate these toxins, it stores them in your fat cells. Eventually these toxins are released from your fat cells, into the bloodstream and so into the brain, lungs, heart, eyes, stomach, liver, etc.

Sugar Is Pro-Inflammatory

Sugar is highly inflammatory in its own right, as well as being a component of manufactured foods, which also ignite "fire in the belly".

Get rid of sugar; it will kill you if you don't. You'll soon lose your "sweet tooth". After a couple of weeks without added sugar, even a carrot will begin to taste very sweet.

Plant substitutes like Stevia are probably non-inflammatory. But I generally tell patients to avoid these products, as they are much sweeter even than sugar and simply keep that sweet tooth going. Better not!

Patients on a diet called the FODMAP diet (avoiding: fermentable, oligosaccharides, disaccharides, monosaccharides, and polyols) did well against gut inflammation.

These sugars are found in wheat, rye, onion, garlic, leeks, artichokes, mushrooms, cauliflower, snow peas, beans, chickpeas, lentils, milk products except hard cheese, honey, apples, pears, watermelon, mangos, stone fruits, high-fructose corn syrup, sorbitol, mannitol, maltitol, and xylitol. And more.

So avoiding those is going to improve a great many people, right? In fact it's a rather severe elimination diet. Although the allowed foods included bananas, blueberries, grapes, oranges, tomatoes, maple syrup, gluten-free breads and cereals, rice noodles and rice, water crackers, oats, polenta, broccoli, bok choy, carrot, cucumber, green beans, sweet potato, olives, lactose-free milk, rice milk, hard cheeses, butter, margarine, and soy yogurt.

What happened was the researchers dumped the patients on this diet for over a year (ugh!) About three quarters got better.

The trouble is, because they don't know how to do this properly, they never follow through. That means to re-introduce banned foods, one at a time, and figure out which are the chief offenders. THOSE are the foods to avoid. Go back and read chapter 9 if you haven't already done so.

[SOURCE: American College of Gastroenterology's 76th Annual Scientific Meeting, Washington D.C., Oct. 28-Nov. 2, 2011].

> Get rid of sugar;
> it will kill you
> if you don't.

All starches are digested into some form of sugar and so are best avoided. They say complex carbohydrates, like polysaccharides, are slower to digest and do not provoke the insulin rush (hungry, then tired after a sugar meal). Some of these are good pre-biotics (page 131). But that's all for naught if you are intolerant of grains and most people are because they are not natural hunter-gatherer foods.

Avoid or keep to a minimum.

Fiber Facts From Fiction

I remember an English comedian (Jasper Carrot) talking about Audrey Eyton's "F-Plan Diet", back in the 1980s. Beans for breakfast, beans for lunch, beans for supper, beans with everything… No wonder it's called the F-Plan, he laughed! (farting, get it?)

I used to joke that if fiber was all it took, we'd just need to chop up the carpets and eat those and we'd all be healthy. I thought there must be more to it than that… And so there is.

If you are confused by it all, you won't be after reading this. Dietary fiber has been a much misunderstood nutrient. Many people know it is important, but not much more than that. It's time to straighten it all out and make it nice and simple.

What Is Fiber?

Dietary fiber, also known as roughage or bulk, includes all parts of plant foods that your body can't digest or absorb. Unlike other food components, such as fats, proteins or carbohydrates, fiber isn't digested by your body. Instead, it passes relatively intact through your stomach, small intestine, colon and out of the other end.

Fiber helps to maintain a solid formed stool, instead of just spludge from your back passage or—even worse—concreted, hard rocks that you can pass only with extreme difficulty.

So it's a part of the process of stool formation but not involved in the carbs, proteins and fats digestion story. Actually, my joke about eating carpets comes close to how you need to picture this.

So what? You might ask. Well, actually fiber is important in many ways, we have discovered over the years. It helps with weight loss, lowers cholesterol, prevents heart disease, lessens the risk of cancer and diabetes, improves digestion and greatly benefits our gut flora, for a start.

Most important of all, fiber quenches inflammation and directly subdues "fire in the belly". It probably absorbs toxins from the gut lumen and that is at least part of the successful anti-inflammatory mechanism.

Pay attention, this is important!

Soluble vs. Insoluble Fiber

There are two main types of fiber: soluble and insoluble. Soluble fiber dissolves in water; insoluble fiber does not. Both are beneficial for health but each in different ways.

Soluble fiber attracts water and forms a gel, which slows down digestion. Soluble fiber delays the emptying of your stomach and makes you feel full, which helps control weight. Slower stomach emptying may also affect blood sugar levels and have a beneficial effect on insulin sensitivity, which may help control diabetes. Soluble fibers can also help lower LDL ("bad") blood cholesterol by interfering with the absorption of dietary cholesterol.

Sources of soluble fiber: oatmeal, oat cereal, lentils, apples, oranges, pears, oat bran, strawberries, nuts, flaxseeds, beans, dried peas, blueberries, psyllium, cucumbers, celery, and carrots.

Insoluble fibers are considered gut-healthy fiber because they have a laxative effect and add bulk to the diet, helping prevent constipation. These fibers do not dissolve in water, so they pass through the gastrointestinal tract relatively intact, and speed up the passage of food and waste through your gut. Insoluble fibers are mainly found in whole grains and vegetables.

Sources of insoluble fiber: whole wheat, whole grains, wheat bran, corn bran, seeds, nuts, barley, couscous, brown rice, bulgur, zucchini, celery, broccoli, cabbage, onions, tomatoes, carrots, cucumbers, green beans, dark leafy vegetables, raisins, grapes, fruit, and root vegetable skins.

Some plants contain significant amounts of both soluble and insoluble fiber. For example plums and prunes have insoluble fiber in the skin and soluble fiber in the pulp.

Synthetic Fiber Products

You probably know about psyllium husks, loved by doctors because it is a "real" drug and prescribable! They like Inulin too, because it's "real" (see below).

There are some other odd products on the market, such as glucomannan, an extract of the konjac plant (also known as konjaku, konnyaku, or the konnyaku potato). It is a water-soluble mixture of glucose and mannose and is considered a fiber product.

Japanese shirataki noodles (also marketed as "miracle noodles") are made from glucomannan. You can put these gooey noodles with anything and assume them to be zero calories. They lack flavor though.

In one 2007 study of glucomannan, published in the British Journal of Nutrition [Br J Nutr. 2008 Jun;99(6):1380-7. Epub 2007 Nov 22.], participants taking a glucomannan and psyllium husk combination supplement lost approximately 10 pounds in 16 weeks compared to 1.7 pounds lost in the placebo group. Another study using only glucomannan showed an average of 5.5 pounds lost over eight weeks, without making any other diet or lifestyle changes [Int J Obes. 1984;8(4):289-93].

Vegetable gum fiber supplements are also relatively new to the market. Often sold as a powder, vegetable gum fibers dissolve easily with no aftertaste. In preliminary clinical trials, they have proven effective for the treatment of irritable bowel syndrome.[Dig Dis Sci. 47 (8): 1697–704] Examples of vegetable gum fibers are guar gum and acacia Senegal gum.

How Much?

We need about 30 – 40 grams a day; women somewhat less than men and we all need less as we grow older. Most Westerners get 20 grams or less: not enough.

But don't suddenly up your intake, otherwise you will be blowing off (breaking wind) and upsetting those around you. Increase your intake slowly towards the optimum and take plenty of water at the same time; soluble fiber needs that and despite what you have read, it isn't easy to pass soluble fiber, if water is short. It will swell and tend to block the intestine, which is the opposite of what is wanted.

As I said, most plants contain both soluble and insoluble fiber. However, the amount of each type varies in different plant foods. If you focus on eating a healthy diet rich in fruits, vegetables, whole grains, legumes, nuts, and seeds, you will certainly take in plenty of fiber.

Remember, animals, fowl and fish foods contain no worthwhile fiber.

Weight Loss Benefits

One of the great things about eating fiber is it gives that pleasant full feeling, without actually adding to your calories. High-fiber foods generally require more chewing, which gives your body time to register when you're no longer hungry, so you're less likely to overeat.

In conjunction with leaving you feeling more satisfied, fiber helps properly regulate our weight-control hormones, such as insulin, ghrelin and leptin. Fiber foods can slow the absorption of sugar and help improve blood sugar levels. So a healthy diet that includes fiber may reduce the risk of developing type 2 diabetes.

Slimmer's need to understand the importance of fiber foods and choose carefully from among them. Fruits and veggies enjoy no great reputation but plant foods are essential for the fiber ingredient they bring.

Pre-Biotics vs. Probiotic

Now we come to the real reason that fiber is important to health. I believe this part of the story is much more relevant than just the idea of chopped up carpets! Fiber is a pre-biotic.

Definition: a pre-biotic is a non-digestible food ingredient that stimulates the healthy growth and/or activity of bacteria in the digestive system in ways beneficial to overall health. The term (and concept) was coined by Marcel Roberfroid in 1995.[J Nutr. 125 (6): 1401–1412]

The prebiotic definition does not emphasize a specific bacterial group. Generally, however, it is assumed that a prebiotic should increase the number and/or activity of bifidobacteria and lactic acid bacteria. The importance of the bifidobacteria and the lactic acid bacteria (LABs) is that these groups of bacteria may have several beneficial effects on the host, especially in terms of improving digestion (including enhancing mineral absorption[J Nutr. 137 (11 Suppl): 2527S–2533S]) and the effectiveness and intrinsic strength of the immune system.[J Nutr. 137 (11 Suppl): 2563S–2567S]

Later you will read that Lactobacillus rhamnosus is one of the best established probiotics, even though it is not a native of our intestines and can, in extreme situations, be a pathogen. The most famous strain is L. rhamnosus lcr35.

Both types of fiber benefit healthy bowel flora but more so the soluble type.

Traditional dietary sources of pre-biotics include soybeans, inulin sources (such as Jerusalem artichoke, jicama, and chicory root), raw oats, unrefined (whole) wheat, unrefined barley, and yacon.

It is interesting to note that the ONLY non-plant source of suitable pre-biotic oligosaccharides is human breast milk and these are believed to play an important role in the development of a healthy immune system in infants.

[Jackson, Frank. "Breast Milk". Jackson GI Medical. http://www.prebiotin.com/breast-milk/ Retrieved 16 June 2013]

Omega-3s

This class of nutrients, called essential fatty acids are remarkable against inflammation. There are countless studies showing they protect against heart disease, diabetes, Alzheimer's etc.

Omega-3s DHA and EPA reduce triglycerides, which can lead to blocked arteries. And omega-3s can also help decrease risk of irregular heartbeats.

Among the Inuit (eskimos), who consume vast quantities of omega-3s in fish and seals blubber etc. Western degenerative diseases - all of which are inflammatory in character - are pretty much unknown. That is, until the Inuit move into the land bases and started eating the Western-type junk diet, rich in omega-6s. You see, omega-6s compete with and displace healthy omega-3 fatty acids.

Omega-6s are highly pro-inflammatory. They occur in vast quantities in typical manufactured foods. But beware: farmed fish, such as tilapia, can have a omega-6 content higher than that of your typical donut!

Trace the omega-6s in your diet and eliminate or reduce them. You'll pick up the small amount you need anyway. This will do a great deal to extinguish inflammation.

Sources of Omega-3s

These include walnuts, which are an excellent source of alpha-linolenic acid (ALA), one of the three main omega-3 fatty acids and the one most commonly found in plants. Other nuts, including pecans and pistachios, also contain ALA, but almonds do not.

Omega-3-enhanced eggs are widely available in stores and farmers markets. They tend to have darker yolks than regular eggs. The omega-3 fatty acid DHA is found in yolks only; egg whites contain no fatty acids, so those "healthy" omelet's made only of egg whites are trash.

Cold-water fish has the highest concentration of DHA and EPA, the two fatty acids closely linked to heart health. The American Heart Association recommends at least two servings per week of salmon, tuna, herring, lake trout, sardines, and similar fish.

Seaweed too, contains lots of omega-3s. Sushi anyone?

There is ALA in leafy green vegetables, but only when fresh.

Now the two main sources:
1. Flaxseeds, Flaxseed Oil, and Other Seeds
2. Best of all: grass-fed beef.

Get Mushrooms!

Here's a little-known secret for reducing inflammation: mushrooms and fungi. This kingdom of living organisms helps in many ways and will intelligently modulate the immune system, helping boost it when needed and helping tone it down when the immune response (inflammation) is excessive.

We call this a biological response modifier (BRM) or adaptogen. Fungi contain hundreds of chemical compounds that are adaptogens. We are discovering more and more of them, all the time. There are around 100 such useful compounds in the Reishi mushroom alone.

Adaptogens engage the immune system is a smart way, instead of all-out suppression, as most anti-inflammatory drugs do (aspirin, Ibuprofen, NSAIDs etc.).

Technically, the adaptogens are terpenes. These substances are resins and found in trees and other plants, as well as fungi, which of course are not in the plant kingdom at all.

These terpenes have great powers to reduce swelling, redness and pain, improve breathing and reduce the first stages of heart disease. That makes them ideal for quelling "Fire In The Belly".

King of the anti-inflammatory mushrooms is the amazing Ganoderma lucidum mushroom; Chinese name Reishi.

In one scientific test, comparing the effects of Reishi to that of hydrocortisone, a simple hot water extract of the fruiting body was every bit as good as the drug. But there were none of the notorious side effects of the corticosteroid drug (immune suppression, water retention, stomach ulcers, etc.)

Here's a short list of useful anti-inflammatory mushrooms:

Hericium erinacous (Lion's mane)

Inonotus obliquus (Chaga mushroom)

Polyporus umbellatus (The umbrella polypore; Chinese Zhuling)

Ganoderma lucidum (Reishi, lingzhi)

Note: There are many useful species in the Ganoderma family.

Other Useful Adaptogens

Adaptogens are herbs which appear to increase the body's ability to adapt to stress and biological change.

The concept of an adaptogen was originally created by the pharmacologist A.V. Lazarev in 1947 to describe novel effects of dibazol 12-benzyl benzimidazol, an arterial dilator developed in France. This concept was later (in the former Soviet Union) applied to describe remedies that increase the resistance of organisms to stress in experimental and clinical studies. According to the original definition adaptogens are non-specific remedies that increase resistance to a broad spectrum of harmful factors "stressors" of different physical, chemical and biological natures.

This definition has been updated and today adaptogens are defined as a "new class of metabolic regulators which increase the ability of an organism to adapt to environmental factors and to avoid damage from such factors."

In spite of an extensive amount of research in the USSR, (by 1984, more than 1,500 pharmacological and clinical published studies), the concept was not generally recognized in Western medicine as it seemed to be in contrast to some of the key-concepts of modern pharmacology: potency, selectivity and the "active ingredient" model, with efficacy balanced by and accepted level of toxicity.[2][3]

In 1998, however, the term adaptogen was allowed officially as a functional claim for certain products by the FDA and by the European Medicines Agency and EFSA.

To be useful, it is said, an adaptogen should exhibit three main traits:

1. It must be nontoxic to the user, at least in any reasonable amount
2. It must also generate a nonspecific response
3. It must help to create a state of balance or normalization in the patient, restoring the natural homeostasis of his or her body

Not only do they help us to cope with stress and the hassles of everyday living, but they are also powerful antioxidants and biological response modifiers (BRMs).

Examples which you can research and source for yourself, either in local health food stores, or on the Internet, include: Chlorella, Maitake Mushroom, Aloe Vera, Rhodiola rosea, Eleutherococcus and Schizandra chinensis.

Don't fall for the "active ingredient" trap. These plants work best when taken whole. We simply do not know enough about the make chemicals to make decisions about what might be the key ingredient. Indeed, it is most unlikely that there is just one key ingredient. It's most likely an orchestra of chemical compounds that produce their remarkable effects.

[SOURCE: Wikipedia]

Herbs Against Inflammation

Lots of natural plant substances seem to have the benefit of calming inflammation in our bodies.

Green Tea

Here we go again with our old friend green tea. But it's true; it is an anti-inflammatory. Studies show that epigallocatechin-3-gallate (EGCG) inhibits the expression of the gene which codes for Interleukin-8, a proinflammatory cytokine.

Take 1- 2 cups a day!

Camomile Tea

Chamomile a plant which belongs to the family of sunflowers has natural anti-inflammatory properties. It contains antioxidants from flavonoids, such as quercetin and luteolin, and chamazulene(an essential oil).

It's also sleep-inducing.

2- 3 cups a day.

Ginkgo Biloba

Here's a surprise. But actually Ginkgo biloba is a putative antioxidant and has been used for thousands of years to treat a variety of ailments, including inflammatory disorders.

Lots or studies form orthodox medicine support this. Here's one from 2008 I found on PubMed.

[Carcinogenesis. 2008 September; 29(9): 1799–1806]

The effect is due, at least in part, to the terpines in Gingko. The ginkgolides inhibit the activity of the compound known as platelet-activating factor (PAF). PAF reduces inflammation by increasing permeability of blood vessels and contracting various involuntary muscles such as those in airways. PAF activation is also associated with the aggregation of platelets, which aid in blood clotting. Ginkgo supplementation has therefore been associated with anti-inflammatory effects as well as reduced blood clotting.

Because of its anti-inflammatory effect Gingko has been proposed for Alzheimer's. Here is a study which reported that G. biloba was able to protect nerve cells exposed to various free radicals.

[Oyama, et al. "Ginkgo biloba extract protects brain neurons against oxidative stress induced by hydrogen peroxide." Brain Research. 1996; 712:349-352]

Beware the anti-platelet factor, which may extend clotting time and be dangerous to those taking anti-coagulants.

Frankincense

Boswellia (Boswellia serrata). Also known as Indian frankincense, Boswellia serrata has long been recognized in Ayurvedic medicine for its anti-inflammatory benefits. Today scientists studying extracts of boswellia report that it can switch off key cell signalers and pro-inflammatory mediators known as cytokines in the inflammatory cascade.

Ginger (Zingiber officinalis)

Valued for centuries the world over for its medicinal qualities, ginger today is being studied by biochemists and pharmacologists interested in its analgesic, anti-inflammatory, anti-nausea, and sugar-moderating effects in the body. In the past 30 years or so their work has confirmed how ginger shares properties with conventional over-the-counter and prescription NSAID's, in that it suppresses the synthesis in the body of the pro-inflammatory prostaglandins (page 32), but with few if any side effects.

Turmeric (Curcuma longa)

Turmeric is an ancient culinary spice native to South East Asia, has been used as an anti-inflammatory agent for centuries in Indian Ayurvedic medicine. Also known as cucurmin, it is a mild COX-2 inhibitor, but works differently from the prescription-strength drugs that can increase your risk of myocardial infarction or stroke.

Zyflamend, from New Chapter, Inc., includes a number of anti-inflammatory herbs, including holy basil, another Indian remedy.

Other anti-inflammatory plants, including spices, are:
- Black Pepper
- Cinnamon
- Rosemary
- Basil
- Cardamon
- Chives
- Cilantro
- Cloves
- Garlic
- Parsley

Arnica montana

Arnica is a widely used homeopathic and/or herbal remedy for inflammation in addition to a salve for bruises & sprains.

Licorice

Licorice root is an effective, natural anti-inflammatory herb root (active ingredient glycyrrhizin). But it's quite toxic and is definitely not a first choice. Note that long-term use can raise blood pressure and lead to potassium loss. Dose is one-eighth to one-quarter teaspoon of extract up to three times daily.

St. John's Wort

This plant is perhaps better known for its antidepressant effect, but also an herbal remedy for inflammation. Follow label directions.

Willow

White willow bark (Salix alba) is also anti-inflammatory and pain-relieving. It's logical, it's related to aspirin and its scientific name gave us the chemical name (salicylic acid).

Fruit enzymes

Bromelain is an anti-inflammatory enzyme from pineapple, so eat lots of fresh pineapple. You can also buy chewable bromelain tablets. Papain from papaya is similar. But a far better idea is a powerful compounding of this and other enzymes from Germany, known as Wobenzym.

Wobenzym

This is one of the most powerful anti-inflammatory compounds I know of. It literally "digests" or eats up circulating inflammatory complexes.

Ingredients include pancreatic enzymes (trypsin, chymotrypsin, lipase and amylase), papain, bromelain, and rutin, a bioflavonoid known to strengthen the smallest blood vessels & help prevent hemorrhage from high blood pressure.

Wobenzym is manufactured by the internationally recognized leader in enzyme preparations, Wobe-Mucos of Germany. It has been tested, researched, utilized and prescribed by medical professionals like me for over forty years. It's proven!

The enzymes in this preparation act as a "biological vacuum cleaner" eliminating impurities, foreign proteins, immune complexes and harmful micro-organisms from the blood stream and tissues. This greatly diminishes the inflammatory response and allows the normal immune functions to operate at a much healthier level.

Wobenzym is far safer than anti-inflammatory drugs, such as Ibuprofen or NSAIDs.

Recommended use: 2-3 tablets, 2-3 times daily, on an empty stomach, 45 minutes before meals.

Dosages as high as 10 tablets, 3 times daily may be used in serious cases.

Avoid during pregnancy and seek careful monitoring if you take anti-coagulant medication.

Vitamins and Minerals

As well as herbs, you need to bear in mind that many vitamins and minerals are anti-inflammatory. Indeed, they probably all are, since tissue damage results from any nutritional lack and that in turn will lead inevitably to inflammation.

Vitamin D is a powerful anti-inflammatory.

Studies have shown that supplementation with relatively high doses (50 mcg daily for 9 months) is able to significantly increase the anti-inflammatory cytokine IL-10 by over 40% and relatively decrease or block an increase in the dangerous pro-inflammatory cytokine TNF-alpha.

Vitamin A

A 2008 paper by scientists in the Molecular Immunology and Inflammation Branch at the National Institute of Arthritis and Musculoskeletal and Skin Diseases (NIAMS) showed how retinoic acid signaling can promote or suppress the activity of helper T cells, a class of immune cells involved in inflammatory responses.

A balance between two kinds of helper T cells - pro-inflammatory Th17 cells and anti-inflammatory T regulatory cells – is essential to avoid over-activity of the immune system, which could result in inflammation and autoimmune diseases.

Helper T cells play a critical role in the delicate balance between the immune system's normal defense of the body from infection and immune system overactivity, which results in mistaken attacks on the body's own cells and can sometimes produce autoimmune disease.

Retinoic acid, a byproduct of vitamin A, appears to promote the production of the anti-inflammatory T regulatory cells. This was further confirmed by the fact that using an inhibitor of retinoic acid reduced the production of T regulatory cells.

[Elias K, et al. Retinoic acid inhibits Th17 polarization and enhances FoxP3 expression through a Stat-3/Stat-5 independent signaling pathway. Blood 2008;111:1013-1020]

> Retinoic acid, a byproduct of vitamin A, appears to promote the production of the anti-inflammatory T regulatory cells.

We need at least 1,000 units daily; 2,000 is better. But by convention, women are warned this could harm a pregnancy (even though LACK of vitamin A leads to spina bifida deformity: go figure).

Vitamin E

Vitamin E is an antioxidant that decreases inflammation, rebuilds damaged joints and tissues, soothes irritated and inflamed tissues, hydrates the body, heals wounds and lowers your risk of inflammatory diseases such as arthritis, Alzheimer's disease, lupus, inflammatory bowel disease, asthma and allergies

Selenium quenches free radicals.

This is straight form a paper on PubMed and says it all:

The essential trace element selenium (Se), in the form of selenoproteins, plays a pivotal role in the antioxidant defense system of the cell. There is evidence that Se may confer benefits in patients with inflammatory disease and even infectious diseases like HIV. Furthermore, in patients with severe sepsis, characterized by an increase in reactive oxygen species and low endogenous anti-oxidative capacity, as well as in patients with systemic inflammatory response syndrome, Se supplementation may reduce mortality and improve the clinical outcome, respectively.

[Horm Metab Res. 2009 Jun;41(6):443-7. Epub 2009 May 5]

100 mcg a day is minimum. Strive for 200 mcg daily and hang the expense. Selenium also protects against mercury poisoning and against cancer, so don't even think about it. Take it.

Magnesium

Magnesium is enormously powerful at cooling the "fire" of inflammation. Yet it is the commonest mineral deficiency in our diets. The majority of people are not coming anywhere near the RDA minimum of 350 mg.

Researchers from the Medical University of South Carolina measured blood inflammation levels–using the C-reactive protein (CRP) test–in 3,800 men and women. The shocking finding was that many people were getting less than the RDA: 50% less! These individuals were almost three times as likely to have dangerously high CRP levels as those who consumed enough. Being over age 40 and overweight and consuming less than 50% of the RDA more than doubled the risk of blood vessel-damaging inflammation.

[http://www.prevention.com/cda/article/magnesium-chills-inflammation/
9c9150d1fa803110VgnVCM10000013281eac_____/health/healthy.living.centers/heart.conditions]

146

The fact is magnesium is crucial to the inflammatory process. Increases in extracellular magnesium concentration cause a decrease in the inflammatory response and vice versa: reduction in the extracellular magnesium results in more inflammation. It's proven. So if you want to live longer and avoid the inflammatory diseases of aging, including deadly heart attacks (coronary occlusion events), make sure you take adequate magnesium daily.

[Magnesium and inflammation: lessons from animal models] Clin Calcium. 2005 Feb;15(2):245-8. Review. Japanese. PMID: 15692164
[PubMed - indexed for MEDLINE]

According to Dr. Sophie Begona, magnesium-deficient rats develop a generalized inflammation.

[Assessment of the relationship between hyperalgesia and peripheral inflammation in magnesium-deficient rats. Sophie Begona, Abdelkrim Allouia, Alain Eschaliera, André Mazurb, Yves Rayssiguierb and Claude Dubray, Pharmacologie Fondamentale et Clinique de la Douleur, Laboratoire de Pharmacologie Médicale, Faculté de Médecine, France]

Dr. Andrzej Mazura and team at Milan University confirmed that magnesium modulates cellular events involved in inflammation. Experimental magnesium deficiency in the rat induces, after only a few days, a clinical inflammatory syndrome characterized by leukocyte and macrophage activation, release of inflammatory cytokines and acute phase proteins; and excessive production of free radicals. Increase in extracellular magnesium concentration, decreases inflammatory response while reduction in the extracellular magnesium results in cell activation.

[Magnesium and the inflammatory response: Potential physiopathological implications. Andrzej Mazura, Jeanette A.M. Maierb, Edmond Rocka, Elyett Gueuxa, Wojciech Nowackic and Yves Rayssiguiera. University of Milan, Department of Preclinical Sciences, Milan, Italy]

In other words you cannot afford to be deficient in magnesium; it kick starts the whole inflammatory process, with all the attendant dangers I have been writing about.

To protect yourself, take a minimum of 350 mg daily. Double that is better and will overcome any disposition towards malabsorption.

Chapter 11 Heavy Metal Toxicity

I have hinted that toxic heavy metals, like lead and mercury, are bowel inflammatory. Indeed they are and they form part of a complex inflammatory issue which needs vigorous quenching.

"The fact is that all metals are toxic

Toxic heavy metals are intended by Nature to be excreted into the gut, via the liver and bile secretions. But the inflammatory process which is set up as a result causes "leaky gut syndrome", a condition in which inappropriate substances are absorbed from the intestines and put back into the metabolic pathways.

This includes heavy metals. So they are re-absorbed and have to go through the liver a second, third and fourth time, over and over, as the body struggles to get rid of this enormous inflammatory burden.

Each time this happens, our most crucial detox molecule, glutathione, gets used up and is not recovered. Thus, to detox heavy metals safely we need very large amounts of glutathione, to replenish the molecules lost in this way.

It's hard to supplement glutathione orally but, luckily, taking so-called precursor substances, such as alpha lipoic acid and N-acetyl cysteine help provoke manufacture of glutathione.

The section on heavy metal toxicity which follows is from a much-loved article on the Internet. You can also hear me talking it through on radio at:

http://www.alternative-doctor-radio.com

Obviously, heavy metal toxicity is not confined merely to the bowel but it concerns us greatly here. I have been writing for over 30 years that the commonest cause of intractable infections, especially dysbiosis, Candida etc., is heavy metal poisoning the immune system.

Many people have become aware of the mercury toxicity problem. But it would be a mistake to think that metal poisoning is unique to this particular toxin. Consider: silver colloid is an antiseptic and has been used since ancient times to inhibit bacteria in drinking water. If it poisons germs, it will poison you. I have written elsewhere in the site that iron forms the most destructive free-radical of all ("hot iron"), very damaging to life.

The fact is that *all metals are toxic* and our bodies require special transport and handling mechanisms to keep them from harming us. This applies just as much as essential minerals, like iron, zinc and chromium, as it does to non-essential metals and metalloids, like cadmium and arsenical compounds.

Heavy Metals And Cancer

Metals can directly and indirectly damage DNA and that means an increased risk of cancer (we call this genotoxicity). There are also possibly non-genotoxic pathways, due to irritation or immuno-toxicity. Sure enough, a number of metals are known to be carcinogenic. These are:

> arsenic and arsenic compounds,
>
> beryllium and beryllium compounds,
>
> cadmium and cadmium compounds,
>
> nickel compounds and
>
> hexavalent chromium (remember the movie "Erin Brockovich"?)

The usual target is the lung, though arsenic has a unique association with skin cancers that has been recognized for many years.

It is a fact that metal implants in the body (as, for example, in bone pinning or plates) may be associated with adjacent cancers, caused by irritation of the tissues. The late Patrick Stortebecker at the Karolinska Institute in Stockholm also pointed out the frequency with which cancer of the jaw was found in association with metal amalgam fillings. That is disturbing, since this particular kind of "prosthetic" tends to be very long term and very common indeed.

A major development in dentistry is the titanium implant, to replace lost teeth. But it is an act of faith to suppose that titanium is inert.

The presence of toxic metals in our systems is highly significant for they are capable of causing serious health problems through interfering with normal biological functioning. Although they can be found in high concentrations in the body, a number of these heavy metals (aluminum, beryllium, cadmium, lead and mercury) have no known biological function. Others (arsenic, copper, iron and nickel) are thought to be essential at low concentrations, but are toxic at high levels. Generally speaking, heavy metals disrupt metabolic function in two basic ways:

> First, they accumulate and thereby disrupt function in vital organs and glands such as the heart, brain, kidneys, bone, liver, etc.

> Second, they displace vital nutritional minerals from where they should be in the body to provide biological function. For example, enzymes are catalysts for virtually every biochemical reaction in all life-sustaining processes of metabolism. But instead of calcium being present in an enzyme reaction, lead or cadmium may be there in its place. Toxic metals can't fulfill the same role as the nutritional minerals, thus their presence becomes critically disruptive to enzyme activity.

Because their impact is at such a foundational level, heavy metals can be causal factors in literally any health problem.

If your job or living circumstances expose you to heavy metals, you would do well to minimize or eliminate your exposure as much as possible. Be aware that there are many ways these toxins can be absorbed into your body--through foods and beverages, skin exposure, and via the air you breathe. So, whenever possible, wear gloves, use protective breathing apparatuses, and be sure to obtain fresh air ventilation.

Persistence In The Environment

One of the problems with metals is their environmental persistence. Once mined and brought into the ecology, they last almost indefinitely.

Also, we face the usually-ignored problem of potentiation, which means two relatively small doses of two different substances may have a dramatically enhanced effect when present together. For instance it is not widely known that the presence of lead (which is everywhere) makes mercury 100 times more toxic.

We call these metal-metal interactions and they might be quite critical in the formation of cancers. Animal studies also indicate, for example, that calcium enhances lead toxicity in rats and cadmium increases the likelihood of cadmium-induced prostatic cancer.

Given these insights, the complacency of traditional dentists over the cocktail of metalloids they put in our mouths as "amalgam" is little short of scientific folly. In the US they call them silver fillings, in an effort to imply purity and divert from the fact they are an amalgam of several different metals, of which silver is only a small proportion of the whole.

Protection From Other Metals

But it also works the other way, fortunately. The presence of a second metal may actually protect against toxicity. Thus, for instance, magnesium was shown in animal studies to prevent cadmium-induced testicular tumors and zinc blocks lung cancer caused by continued inhalation of cadmium. Both magnesium and manganese were effective at preventing tumors which otherwise formed at the site of nickel injections in rats.

In fact magnesium has been shown to have a wide variety of beneficial effects against metal carcinogenesis risk factors. It is yet another reason why magnesium is one of the most vital and health-giving nutrients we have. Avoid deficiency at all costs.

150

Also, we have known for decades that selenium is vitally protective against mercury and also has a powerful anti-cancer benefit. When the daily intake is 100 mcg or more (200 mcg is better), the risk of cancer from all sources drops dramatically.

Avoiding Heavy Metal Exposure Is Impossible

Preventative measures are worthwhile and important, but ultimately futile. The inescapable reality is that it is impossible in this day and age not to be exposed to heavy metals. It is only a matter of how much and how often.

Apart from living in isolation on a organic farm, not much. And that's only relative. Don't be fooled that you would be safe in this environment; metals are in the air, as experience with strontium 90 and other radio-active atoms shows. Attempts to remove lead from our motor combustion engines is a good start. Better copper-based plumbing, is also a right move.

But there is much pollution in the food chain. Lead dust is everywhere by the highways and in the dirt, left there from over a quarter of a century ago, when it was spewed by motor exhausts. Having an intelligent strategy to get rid of heavy metal poisons is critical to survival in the coming century and much wiser than wishing it wasn't there or wanting to run away to some transient utopia.

So we need to get rid of this killer junk. What can we do? Reduce exposure by all means possible.

But rely more on competitive inhibition: that means the presence of "good" metals to squeeze out the bad ones. Remember all metals are toxic. But in reasonable physiological doses zinc, magnesium and selenium are important protective's. Fill up the seats with good guys and the bad guys can't enjoy the show.

You should be taking 200 mcg. daily of selenium, 20- 50 milligrams of zinc (citrate form is shown to be best absorbed) and 350 milligrams of magnesium, as the orotate, gluconate or amino-chelate. Watch out for diarrhea from magnesium salts, otherwise you might actually suffer a loss of mineral intake.

> "Lead dust is everywhere by the highways and in the dirt, left there from over a quarter of a century ago, when it was spewed by motor exhausts."

These will tend to squeeze the bad guys.

But the final answer is chelation. Chelation means, by definition, grasping and eliminating heavy metal poisons. It's a whole subject in itself.

Chelation

DMPS, DMSA, Kelmer and EDTA. Where the situation is serious, for example, lead or copper overload, I give IV ethyldiethylamine tetracetic acid (EDTA), in a series of infusions taking 3 hours or so each. The many benefits of this therapy can be read elsewhere on the Internet.

Unfortunately, this therapy is inadequate for mercury toxicity. There are three effective strategies for mercury, each with pros and cons:

6- 10 IV infusions of DMPS, 3 mgms per kg of body weight. These need skilled experience but done properly and at the correct dose I find have virtually no side-effects. The theoretical risk here is that DMPS crosses the blood-brain barrier and may carry mercury into neurological tissues, where it is most unwelcome. Side effects can be unpleasant and this seems the least advisable method.

Oral DMSA, 30 mgms per kg body weight. Duration depends on response but in the region of 6- 10 weeks. Side effects can be unpleasant but can be ameliorated by reducing the dose. Generally children tolerate DMSA much better than adults.

Oral chelation with magnesium succinate (*marketed as Kelmer), 60 mg per kg body weight. I am satisfied that this produces the same degree of mercury elimination as DMSA but without the unwanted side effects. It just takes longer, that's all!

There is controversy over whether oral EDTA will remove mercury. For all sorts of scientific reasons, to do with valence and electrical charge, it shouldn't work well. But Dr. Garry Gordon claims is does: by actual urine and tissue testing, that it can be seen being excreted after his oral chelation regime (which admittedly includes a lot more than mere EDTA).

Self-administered therapy is not recommended. But chlorella is a great heavy metal attractor, is safe and plentiful. Lesser players are garlic and cilantro.

Finally, remember that once the source of contamination is removed, if you support your body with good detox and nutritional requirements, especially glutathione precursors, the heavy metals will gradually disappear from the tissues by slow attrition, a process termed leaching or, more exactly,

depuration.

Intestinal Metal Detox (IMD)

The best answer to date that I have found for this heavy metal inflammatory overload is Christopher Shade's Intestinal Metal Detox (a proprietary name).

Quicksilver Scientific, Shade's company, has developed a sophisticated detoxification system based on enhancing the natural removal of metals through the intestines using a highly purified silica carrier with covalently attached metal-binding groups.

The product is insoluble and functions by mouth to bind heavy metals in the gut so that they can be safely eliminated with the bowels; this prevents both absorption of the heavy metals and the generation of free-radicals catalyzed by the metals. In fact, the product can also directly neutralize free-radicals in the gut and thus may play a role in damping gastrointestinal inflammation.

Both the silica base and the binding agent are GRAS (generally recognized as safe) for use in food, but since the binding agent is firmly attached to the insoluble silica, it is not absorbed and thus not bioavailable.

The product contains no known allergens and no allergic reactions have been reported to date.

IMD binds mercury and of course other heavy metals in the intestines and escorts these harmful contaminants out of the body. In other words, it breaks the vicious cycle of enterohepatic re-circulation, in which excreted metals cause bowel inflammation, leading to leaky gut and thus reabsorption of the toxins!

It also leads to lowering of blood mercury levels, allowing organ and tissue bound mercury safely to drain into the blood at a natural rate, including brain-bound mercury.

IMD fortifies the link between the intestines and the immune system.

1 scoop mixed in water or juice daily on an empty stomach; take 5 days on and 2 days off in a rotation. Take away from minerals, Glutathione, and Clear Way Cofactors.

For advanced use take 1 scoop, 2-3 times daily. For sensitive patients, start with half a scoop per day, and work up to the full dosage. Children 12 and under: 1/2 scoops, or as tolerated.

Caution: not to be used by infants, pregnant or nursing women.

Dosage: Regimen: For a long-term cleanse take 5 days on/ 2 days off in a rotation. For acute problems, take continuously until symptoms subside.

Length of Treatment: The general course of use is 4-6 months as a basic cleanse, up to a year for deeper cleansing. Periodic use after the main cleanse (one month two times per year) is helpful for two reasons:

1. To remove new accumulations, and

2. Deeper deposits may not be accessible during the first cleanse and can move out and become more available after the body adjusts to the first cleanse.

The speed/intensity of the cleanse can be controlled by the dosage. Most people experience a need for more sleep at night, but if pronounced fatigue is experienced during the day, the dosage can be decreased until comfortable. No major side effects have been reported. Minor side effects include: fatigue and mild headaches. These reactions are common during any type of cleansing. During this cleanse it is important to increase water intake and make sure that you are having at least 1-2 bowel movements a day.

Supply: 6 gram powder (3 month supply) - SRP$150.00

It comes with a pre-measured scoop for easy use.

Obtain IMD from Quicksilver Scientific. You can also find a suitable practitioner to work with, starting from this page:

http://www.quicksilverscientific.com/clinical/the-human-detoxification-system.html

QS Tri-Test

Quicksilver Scientific's Tri-Test is the only clinical testing suite that measures both the exposures and excretion abilities for each of the two main forms of mercury we are exposed to. The QS Tri-Test utilizes mercury speciation analysis, a patented advanced technology that separates methyl mercury from inorganic mercury and measures each directly. This technique provides unprecedented information for the healthcare practitioner to assess the patient's difficulties with each form of mercury and plan a successful detoxification strategy.

The Analytical Suite and Results Reporting

Chapter 12 **Solving Dysbiosis**

You have learned the great menace of letting your natural bowel flora become corrupted, from unwise eating and drinking, lifestyle errors and antibiotic use.

Here's how to get on track for restoring, at least in part, to the state is should be in. The final answer will also include, in part, advice from the next section, so read it too, before writing up your health plan!

There is no question that chow is the key to bowel health. This falls into three principles:

Avoid the foods that the microbiome tells you that you cannot metabolize and handle properly (the older term: food allergens)

Eat plenty of the foods that support the establishment of healthy microbiome patterns (pre-biotics)

Take probiotics. Although these appear not to be such powerful modulators of gut flora and health as the previous two, probiotics definitely help. *Lactobacillus* is now discredited. Not that it's worthless, just not very effective. What you really want is *bacteroides* strains, and human strains at that, exactly as I have been saying in my books since the 1988 *Allergy Handbook*.

Lower Inflammation

Several studies highlighted during a press briefing at the American College of Gastroenterology 2011 Annual Scientific Meeting and Postgraduate Course made it clear that probiotics settle down inflammation.

The researchers hypothesized that microbial imbalance in the gut could explain the present increased incidence of a wide range of inflammatory disorders; it's almost an epidemic. To test whether altering the balance between good and bad bacteria in the gut raises the immune regulatory response, which could lower inflammation, researchers from Cork in Ireland, conducted a double-blind placebo controlled study.

The results were plain enough.

By giving a specific probiotic orally, researchers were able to reduce the levels of these pro-inflammatory cytokines and actually enhance the production of an anti-inflammatory cytokines, to a significant degree.

Plasma levels of the anti-inflammatory cytokine interleukin (IL)-10 rose significantly, while levels of two pro-inflammatory cytokines — tumor necrosis factor-alpha and IL-6 — dropped in all patients who received probiotics.

C-reactive protein level (another big marker for inflammation) was also significantly lower in patients with psoriasis, ulcerative colitis, and chronic fatigue after treatment with the bacterium than after treatment with placebo.

So orthodox medicine has come a long way in the last 20 years. It's almost caught up with doctors like me, who were saying this 20 years ago. I even had it in several of my 1980s books!

[American College of Gastroenterology (ACG) 2011 Annual Scientific Meeting and Postgraduate Course: Abstracts P650, P120, P60, P283. Presented November 1, 2011]

If only they'd listened!

Start By Colon Cleansing

First we need to get rid of the gunk that is backed up in your bowel and then transform and support a healthier bowel flora.

All of the food you eat eventually winds up in your colon. And what your body doesn't use can remain as waste byproducts and toxins. This can cause you to feel bloated, constipated, fatigued, and just plain terrible.

Getting rid of these toxins will help support your immune system, clear your mind, balance your hormones, and markedly reduce inflammation. It will simply help you feel more energetic and healthy.

One of the best ways to get rid of this toxic biological garbage is with a colon cleanse.

A colon cleanse can reduce the level of toxins in your digestive system and reduce inflammation naturally. I'm not in favor of enemas; it's an artificial approach to bowel health and hygiene.

What you put in at the top has far more effect on your health than anything you can wash out at the bottom.

There are several natural ways to get your colon moving and emptying. Simple herbs, such as Cascara, Slippery Elm and Peppermint are good to try.

Cascara Sagrada – This plant extract helps to stimulate the muscles of your colon to contract, helping to push waste out of your body. It also helps strengthen and tone your colon, bringing bowel function back to normal.

Slippery Elm Bark – This herb acts as an "internal soother." It absorbs toxins which can cause intestinal imbalance. It helps stabilize gastritis, diarrhea, irritable bowel syndrome, and even hemorrhoids.

Peppermint Leaf Extract – One of nature's oldest and best tasting natural herbs. Studies have shown that it shortens the time food spends in your stomach. It helps you digest food before it goes into the intestines and colon.

You can find all of these natural herbs in your local health food store. They also come in premixed blends.

Colon Cleanse Preparation

A better idea is a formula I recommend a lot, called Natural Balance. It's from an ancient Persian family recipe, possibly as much as 1,000 years old.

Natural Balance is a safe and easy program to support the digestive system. The following suggestion works well for most people, although it may have to be adjusted to suit your particular needs.

Begin with one capsule of Natural Balance. The herbs can be swallowed as capsules or made into a herbal tea with warm-hot, rather than boiling water. Natural Balance should be taken at night one hour (or more) after supper. Stir the tea to prevent the herbs clumping. The advantage of taking it as a tea is that water helps comfortable detoxification and you are encouraged to drink at least six 8oz. glasses of pure (not distilled) water every day.

Those prone to diarrhea or loose stools might react more immediately to the herbs and may find it helpful to start with half a capsule of Natural Balance each day; those prone to constipation may need to increase the number of capsules until bowel movements come daily.

Anyone with a chemical sensitivity should start with smaller doses of Natural Balance - for example ¼ or ½ a capsule a day and contact us for further guidance.

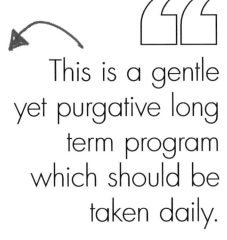

This is a gentle yet purgative long term program which should be taken daily.

The goal, according to the herbalists, is to have at least 2 bowel movements each day. With Natural Balance, if there is no increase in the number of bowel movements within the first three or four days, increase the dosage to two or even three capsules. These can be taken all together. These levels should not be exceeded without contacting www.naturalresources.net or your healthcare practitioner.

Continue for as long as you feel you are benefitting. This is a gentle yet purgative long term program which should be taken daily. Although some people have experienced immediate results do not expect them within the first few days. Be ready to honor any bowel movements quickly as your body becomes used to Natural Balance.

This guide is primarily for teenagers and adults, and not for children under 12.

Suppliers recommend that you do not take any of the products whilst pregnant, nursing or trying for a baby. You should consult your healthcare practitioner if you have frequent diarrhea, abdominal pain, are taking medication or have a medical condition.

Natural Balance Ingredients: Fennel Seed, Psyllium Seed Husk, Rhubarb Root, Peppermint Leaves, Black Seed, Cumin Seed, Cinnamon Stick, Ginger Root.

For more information, or to buy Natural Balance, contact my friend Graeme Dinnen at Resources For Life in England 0800 074 4279 website: www.resourcesforlife.net

Take Probiotics

According to the currently adopted definition by FAO/WHO, probiotics are: "Live microorganisms which when administered in adequate amounts confer a health benefit on the host".

[Report of a Joint FAO/WHO Expert Consultation on Evaluation of Health and Nutritional Properties of Probiotics in Food Including Powder Milk with Live Lactic Acid Bacteria (October 2001)]

Lactic acid bacteria (LAB) and bifidobacteria are the most common types of microbes used as probiotics; but certain yeasts and bacilli may also be used. Probiotics are commonly consumed as part of fermented foods with specially added active live cultures; such as in yogurt, soy yogurt, or as dietary supplements.

The original observation of the positive role played by certain bacteria was first introduced by Russian scientist and Nobel laureate Élie Metchnikoff, who in the beginning of the 20th century suggested that it would be possible to modify the gut flora and to replace harmful microbes with useful microbes. Metchnikoff, at that time a professor at the Pasteur Institute in Paris, proposed the hypothesis that the aging process results from the activity of putrefactive (proteolytic) microbes producing toxic substances in the large bowel. Proteolytic bacteria such as clostridia, which are part of the normal gut flora, produce toxic substances including phenols, indols and ammonia from the digestion of proteins.

It was at that time known that milk fermented with lactic-acid bacteria inhibits the growth of proteolytic bacteria because of the low pH produced by the fermentation of lactose.

Metchnikoff had observed that certain rural populations in Europe, for example in Bulgaria and the Russian steppes, who lived largely on milk fermented by lactic-acid bacteria were exceptionally long lived. Based on these facts, Metchnikoff proposed that consumption of fermented milk would "seed" the intestine with harmless lactic-acid bacteria and decrease the intestinal pH and that this would suppress the growth of proteolytic bacteria.

Metchnikoff himself introduced in his diet sour milk fermented with the bacteria he called "Bulgarian Bacillus" and found his health benefited. Friends in Paris soon followed his example and physicians began prescribing the sour milk diet for their patients.

The rest, as they say, is history. Though ironically, nobody thinks that yogurt is the best way to go, these days. It still works, though.

There are now so many studies showing the clear benefits of taking probiotics that even the orthodox medical community has been won over. But the usual story, that we are populating the gut with "friendly" bacteria may be open to question. Probiotics may help us in other, less direct, ways as suggested by a recent study I found.

The study showed that taking probiotics did not markedly influence the population of organisms at all. But it did alter the digestive function and the individual's tolerance of certain foods.

Here's how it was done. Germ-free mice were carefully raised so that the environment of their guts mimicked that of humans. In effect, the mouse guts played host solely to 15 human gut microbes, all of which had been genetically sequenced.

Next, seven sets of healthy, young-adult human female twins were recruited.

Over four months, the "humanized" mice and the twins consumed a commercially available probiotic-cultured yogurt. The researchers analyzed bacterial gut composition and behavior patterns before, during and after probiotic consumption.

There are now so many studies showing the clear benefits of taking probiotics that even the orthodox medical community has been won over.

The bacterial environment found in the guts of both mouse and man was roughly the same before and after yogurt consumption.

A subsequent urine analysis among the "humanized" mice unearthed "significant changes" in the activity of enzymes involved in metabolism, the team said.

So it may be naïve to think we are populating the gut with "friendly" microbes (maybe not) but it's certainly evidence that probiotics are capable of producing profound changes in the human microbiome function, if not structure.

Justin Sonnenburg, an assistant professor of microbiology and immunology at Stanford University School of Medicine, in California, praised the research as "interesting, subtle and incredibly well-designed."

The study is published in the Oct. 26, 2011, issue of Science Translational Medicine.

Funding for the research came from the U.S. National Institutes of Health (NIH) and Danone Research, an arm of the food conglomerate that makes Dannon probiotic yogurt Activia.

The point is that probiotics are remedies with "vanishingly low side effects," according to Fergus Shanahan, MD, FACG, professor and chair of the Department of Medicine at University College Cork (Ireland).

However, in all the positive enthusiasm for probiotics, a note of caution has been sounded. It might be wise to ask the question: can we ever fully restore bowel flora, once damaged? Or is it permanent? It certainly does not pay to be complacent and make assumptions. Our bowel flora was evolved over millions of years and is not easily replaced or corrected.

In a provocative editorial published this week in Nature, Martin Blaser of New York University's Langone Medical Center argues that antibiotics' impact on gut bacteria is permanent — and so serious in its long-term consequences that medicine should consider whether to restrict antibiotic prescribing to pregnant women and young children.

[Blaser MJ. Stop the killing of beneficial bacteria. Nature 476, 393–394 (25 August 2011). doi:10.1038/476393a]

Taking Yogurt

I have already suggested this may not be the best way to supplement probiotics. But it's certainly the easiest.

TV ads laud the benefits of big commercial products, like Activia , but I'm not convinced by their puff.

The one that does seem to work well as an oral liquid supplement is Yakult (said to be derived from the word "Jahurto", meaning "yogurt" in Esperanto!), developed by Japanese researcher Minoru Shirota. It contains a special bacterium, *Lactobacillus casei Shirota*. Today, Yakult is sold in 31 countries, although its bacteria cultures are provided from a mother strain from Japan regardless of production location.

Note: Yakult contain 18 gr of sugar per 100 mls, which is HIGH (Coca-cola only contains 10 gr sugar per 100 mls).

In general, if you want to use yogurt, look for small manufacturers, who guarantee their product is live. Better still, if you can tolerate milk and want to make your own, get a yogurt maker. One live culture is enough to start you off; then you maintain it by holding back a new "seed" quantity from each batch.

Probiotic Supplements

In theory, these are practical and easy to obtain. In practice, the big problem you have is finding products where the probiotic organisms haven't been killed by the manufacturers processing, such as crushing in a tablet or heating too much.

Make sure you find a product with guaranteed live organisms. You want billions of organisms per capsule. Read the labels and advertising claims.

It makes sense to ask for human strain organisms; for example, the bovine Acidophilus is not nearly as viable in our gut as human strain Acidophilus.

Bifidobacteria actually makes up over 90% of our gut flora, by weight. In the past few years the complete genome sequence of a number of bacterial strains isolated from the human gastrointestinal tract has been established, including that of *Bifidobacterium longum* NCC2705 isolated from the feces of a healthy infant. The ideal product should include plenty of this bacterium.

Probably the number one recognized probiotic in the world today is LCR35, from the acidophilus strain Rhamnosus (Lactobacillus rhamnosus lcr35), created originally by the Society of Warehouses of Roquefort and now manufactured by Lyophyllic Laboratories in Aurillac, in the Cantal region of France. You can find papers on PubMed and NCBI showing its effective absorption and clinical value.

Lactobacillus rhamnosus is a bacterium that was originally considered to be a subspecies of L. casei, but later genetic research found it to be a species of its own. Evidence suggests that it is likely only a transient inhabitant, and not indigenous to the human digestive tract. However is does survive stomach acid and bile and as a great avidity for human intestinal mucosal cells.

Another strain you may come across, marketed with full fanfares blowing, is L. rhamnosus GG. It was patented on 17 April 1985, by Sherwood Gorbach and Barry Goldin, hence the GG from their surnames.

Despite its prestige, L. rhamnosus has appeared as a pathogen on occasion.

[http://en.wikipedia.org/wiki/Lactobacillus_rhamnosus]

Some sources say you must take enteric-coated capsules so that the probiotics will bypass the stomach and stomach acid (which they say destroys the probiotics) and be released in the intestines.

The truth is, natural probiotics are acid and bile resistant. Not only do they pass stomach acid, they implant in the intestine and thrive. Probiotics do not need enteric coating to be effective.

Other food probiotics you might consider include these:

Sauerkraut (fermented cabbage) contains the beneficial microbes leuconostoc, pediococcus, and lactobacillus. Choose unpasteurized sauerkraut because pasteurization (used to treat most supermarket sauerkraut) kills active, beneficial bacteria.

Korean spicy kimchi -- is also loaded with immune-boosting vitamins that may help ward off infection.

Miso. A popular breakfast food in Japan, this fermented soybean paste really can get your digestive system moving. Probiotic-filled miso reportedly contains more than 160 bacteria strains. It's often used to make a salty soup that is low in calories and high in B vitamins and protective antioxidants.

While potentially good for your digestion, not all probiotics can survive the journey through your gastrointestinal tract. But research finds the lactobacillus strains in some fermented soft cheeses, like Gouda, are hardy enough to survive. In addition, cheese may act as a carrier for probiotics which may, in turn, boost the immune system.

Tempeh could work. Made from a base of fermented soybeans, this Indonesian patty produces a type of natural antibiotic that fights certain bacteria. In addition, tempeh is very high in protein. Its flavor has often been described as smoky, nutty, and similar to a mushroom. Tempeh can be marinated and used in meals in place of meat.

Pre-Biotics

I find it interesting that orthodox doctors have led the way with this. There have been many good studies, showing the clear benefits of supporting the colonies of healthy microbes that you are trying to re-establish in the fiery gut.

That can include feeding them and providing fiber as a matrix (a kind of shelter).

Prebiotics are non-digestible food ingredients that stimulate the growth and/or activity of bacteria in the digestive system in ways claimed to be beneficial to health. They were first identified and named by Marcel Roberfroid in 1995.

[Gibson GR, Roberfroid MB. Dietary modulation of the human colonic microbiota: introducing the concept of prebiotics. J Nutr. 1995 Jun;125(6):1401-12. PMID]

Typically, prebiotics are carbohydrates (such as oligosaccharides), but the definition may include non-carbohydrates. The most prevalent forms of prebiotics are nutritionally classed as soluble fiber. To some extent, many forms of dietary fiber exhibit some level of prebiotic effect.

Research now focuses on the distinction between short-chain, long-chain, and full-spectrum prebiotics. "Short-chain" prebiotics, e.g. oligofructose, contain 2-8 links per saccharide molecule, are typically fermented more quickly in the right-side of the colon providing nourishment to the bacteria in that area. Longer-chain prebiotics, e.g. Inulin, contain 9-64 links per saccharide molecule, and tend to be fermented more slowly, nourishing bacteria predominantly in the left-side colon.

So-called full-spectrum prebiotics provide the full range of molecular link-lengths from 2-64 links per molecule, and nourish bacteria throughout the colon.

I don't think it makes sense for the ordinary individual to get involved in this level of complexity. Just eat the stuff!

You can find prebiotics in foods such as asparagus, chicory root*, Jerusalem artichokes*, bananas, oatmeal, red wine, honey, maple syrup, and legumes. Consider eating prebiotic foods on their own or with probiotic foods to perhaps give the probiotics a boost.

* Chicory root and Jerusalem artichoke (completely different plant group to the globe artichoke) are the star prebiotics in my book! The former is 65% prebiotic and the latter 31% (Dandelion greens come in 3rd with 17%). These are figures from the raw vegetable.

Chapter 13 | Deep Tissue Cleansing

This is the "ultimate" anti-inflammatory program, overcoming hidden energetic pathways to inflammation.

Entering the world of electro-acupuncture testing in the mid-1980s was a real eye opener for me. Using this amazing advanced healing modality, we can electrically measure acupuncture meridians for energy, find stressed organs and test for likely toxins and stressors. We can even evaluate remedies by choosing those which get rid of the pathological indicator reads.

> Through electrocupuncture testing I gained breathtaking new insights into the origins of disease.

It's a whole new medical paradigm and I wrote about it in great detail in my book *Virtual Medicine*. You need to read that book to get the full potential of this chapter.

http://www.alternative-doctor.com/virtual_medicine.html

I have mentioned it here as a brief introduction to this chapter, so that you understand, at least in outline, how the information I will be presenting came about.

Through electrocupuncture testing (or EAV, electroacupuncture after Voll, the German researcher who developed it), I gained breathtaking new insights into the origins of disease. I began to work with the concept of a "cascade" effect, in which many factors work one after the other, in a tumbledown effect, finally resulting in symptoms and pathology.

If you can go far back up that cascade, you can work miraculous recoveries by turning off the process, right at cause. Because there were so many real recoveries, it enabled me to be sure that I had found the real cause of the problem.

In this way I began to see that many complex factors led to inflammation and disease. EAV etc., shows us the impact of miasms, old vaccinations, childhood disease, unresolved illness and hidden foci (plural of focus), etc. to create or prolong deep inflammatory processes. We need a means to get them out of the body.

The Focus

One of the key health concepts of EAV is that of a focus. It means a spot in the body that is pathologically altered and is leading to all subsequent symptoms and pathologies. These foci are surprising and varied. For example, hidden dangers in the teeth and jaws lead to a great deal of crippling inflammation elsewhere in the body.

What I called a "hot pelvis", that is, deeply hidden pelvic infections that seem beyond the reach of normal lab tests and the usual antibiotic treatments, is a very common focus found in women who are active sexually.

The key point, obviously, is that if we deal with the focus, the more widespread pathology will quickly resolve.

The Most Stressed Organ

Another key concept seems almost self-explanatory, yet one never meets such a model in conventional medicine. Orthodox doctors are so wrapped up with symptoms and suppressing symptoms, instead of finding true causes, that this approach is outside their field of view altogether (I can't see it therefore it does not exist).

But it's simple. The most stressed organ in the body is obviously *the one which needs healing the most*. But it may have nothing to do with what the patient seems to be suffering from. The complaint may be a skin rash, such as eczema; but the most stressed organ might be the liver. Eczema in fact is often due to what the Chinese and Ayurvedic healers call a "hot liver" (ie. a stressed liver).

Most-stressed organ could be adrenals, parathyroid, pineal or spleen. The pancreas turns up as the most shocked organ many times; something which still needs a satisfactory general model to explain.

Pathology Filters

The next crucial part of the EAV picture is using the electronic detector device to test for WHAT is stressing the organs or WHAT the focus is.

Once again, it is often far removed from what might seem the obvious pathology. For example, glomerulo-nephritis is a kidney inflammation. It's pretty straightforward; until you start using filters. Then you might find that the real cause of the disease is a throat infection from 20 years earlier; or geopathic stress from cell phones; or a childhood vaccination.

I repeat what I said earlier: these strange diagnoses are usually confirmed by the fact that, when you treat them effectively, the patient makes a full recovery! That's all the confirmation that makes sense to me.

Disease stressors can be many and varied. But I have seen triggers as diverse as childhood strep throats, tetanus vaccination (a bad one, that), childhood illnesses, stealth pathogens, jaw erosion and Ascaris (a parasite worm).

Usually, the picture that emerges starts to make sense and the mother of the child, for instance, will start to recall a sequence of illnesses that fits the pattern the EAV is revealing to us. I treated a popular singer once, who had suffered a disastrous stroke. The EAV machine told me the pathology was from a 1986 influenza virus (it's different every year).

He then recalled, vividly, that he had suffered a very debilitating bout of flu that year, which had gone on for weeks and kept him from performing. So I was able to tell him that his stroke had originated over a decade before.

The nice corollary to this is that when I gave him the 1986 flu remedy, he started moving his paralyzed limbs within minutes. A surprising few weeks later, he was back onstage; it would normally have taken him a year to achieve that, if at all.

So How Do We Fix The Various Causes Of Inflammation?

I hinted that, by using EAV devices, we may be able to match a suitable remedy to the disease. It depends what we find. If the focus is a dental abscess, the dentist can fix that.

But most often we resort to a range of remedies which I want to introduce to you now. You'll soon see why this chapter is titled "deep tissue cleansing".

The specialty is called homotoxicology (toxins of the self, literally). It doesn't need to be linked to EAV but all good EAV practitioners are good at homotoxicology.

First, the model it's based on:

Deep Tissue Cleansing

Despite a clumsy name, homotoxicology is a wonderful natural healing modality. It is a therapeutic branch which enables deep cleansing of the body tissues, removing old toxins, disease processes and degenerative debris, leaving the body fluids clean, fresh and able to function as intended.

Based on homeopathy, but not quite the same thing, homotoxicology is the brain child of German doctor Hans-Heinrich Reckeweg (1905-1985). Knowing homeopathy and drawing on a vast knowledge of herbal lore and medicines, he compounded a store of remedies which trod a line between folk medicine and basic plant pharmacology. In the course of time it has proved itself so well that tens of thousands of German doctors use it in daily practice, although less well known in the rest of the world. It has been also called the German system of homeopathy, though this is slightly comical, since the original system of homeopathy was also invented by a German, Samuel Hahnemann.

The Matrix In Health And Disease

Whereas so much molecular medicine is aimed at the cell, as if it were the sole seat of disease, Dr. Alfred Pischinger, then professor of Histology and Embryology in Vienna, saw with great insight that the extracellular fluids, which bathe and feed the cells, were an important key to health.

These fluids, which Pischinger called the "matrix", because it supports everything else, brings nutrition, oxygen, hormone messengers and other vital substances to the tissues and removes excretion products, toxins and the residue of old diseases.

168

Cells may be important but not a separate entity, because they cannot exist without being nurtured in this fluid matrix. Reckeweg pursued Pischinger's matrix model and devised ways to use natural substances to support, clean and revitalize the extracellular matrix. Most of the classic homeopathic remedies are still there, though used slightly differently.

Homeopathic Mixtures

The key variation is the uses of these remedy mixtures, which classic homeopaths frown upon. But Reckeweg ignored the dogma and carried out decades of practical research, demonstrating conclusively that the complex formulations worked and worked well. He made compounds which would support the liver and kidneys, which would work for flu, diabetes, women's problems, stimulate metabolism, tone up the immune system, retard tumors, repair inflammation, act as pain-killers and so on. In other words these are function-based medicines.

The mixtures give rise to yet another name you may encounter "complex homeopathy". Not all remedies are mixtures of substances however; some are single remedies in mixtures of potencies (called a "chord", after the musical term for several notes sounding at once).

- There are key advantages to using potency chords:
- Deeper action
- Fewer initial aggravations than classical dosing
- Doses can be repeated
- Broader spectrum of effect
- No problems selecting the appropriate potency
- No problems in assessing the duration or spectrum of action
- Mixing high and low potencies produces an effect that lies somewhere in between: rapid onset (low potency) and long-lasting action (high potency)
- Faster action
- Potency stages retain their own effects

I used a potency chord of the 1986 flu in the example of the stroke case I gave earlier in this chapter.

Remedy Formulation

To give an instance of this mixture modality and explain it more clearly, let us consider in detail one of Reckeweg's original compounds called Tonsilla compositum. It contains 30 remedies in all, some herbal, some mineral, potentized vitamin C and powerful healing substances called nosodes, which are based on original disease processes but diluted many times (quite safe). In addition there is the "message" or "formula" for healthy key tissues, to help the body get its act together in harmony, as it should be (we call these positive remedies "sarcodes", a term which should not be confused with the disease sarcoidosis).

The full list of ingredients in Tonsilla comp. is as follows:

Healthy Organ Tissue (From Pig)

Lymph glands

Tonsils

Bone marrow

Umbilical cord

Embryo

Spleen

Liver

Hypothalamus

Adrenal gland

Hormones

Thyroxine

Natural cortisone

Nosodes (disease causing agents)

Psorinum-nosode (Black Death)

Fever toxin

Intermediate Catalyst from the Kreb's Cycle (promotes metabolism)

Acidum sarcolacticum (sarcolactic acid)

Herbal Sources

Pulsatilla (wind flower_ Conium maculatum (spotted hemlock)

Gallium aparine (goosegrass)

Echinacea augustifolia (cone-flower)

Aesculus hippocastanum (Horse chestnut)

Dulcamara

Coccus cacti

Gentian

Geranium

Minerals

Calcium phosphate

Kalium stibyltartaricum (antimony potassium tartrate)

Mercurius solubilis (mixture containing essentially mercuroamidonitrate)

Barium carbonicum (barium carbonate)

Sulphur

Vitamin

Acidum ascorbicum (vitamin C)

Herbalists will immediately recognize these herbs and understand their mode of action. Homeopathic potentizing does not alter the known effects of herbs.

The Value Of Symptoms

I have already indicated earlier in this text that inflammation starts as Nature's wise response to a threat. It is to protect us and heal us, not make us sick. It is only when the inflammation goes on too long that it starts being destructive (as when the true cause is not found and quickly eradicated).

So it is, in the homotoxicology model, that we view many "symptoms" as positive and healing.

A sneeze is simply an explosive burst of air, designed to rid us of an irritant in the nasal passages. Similarly, diarrhea and/or vomiting are to throw out food toxins, whether poisons or infective organisms. These symptoms should not be idly suppressed without giving some thought to why they are occurring and, if possible, removing the cause, rather than treating the symptom.

The classic "symptom" of this order is fever. An increase is temperature when an infection is taking place is Nature's solution; not the problem. A fever selectively mobilizes immune cells and favors them over the pathogens. Fever is a good thing and should not be suppressed.

One thing we soon learn from EAV is that if a disease is not allowed to resolve naturally, but is suppressed by medications aimed only at blocking the symptoms, the disease will simply go dormant. It then emerges years, or even decades later, in a far more destructive form.

So, for example, I have seen crippling arthritis in later life caused by childhood illnesses, such as staph and strep, which were suppressed by antibiotics and paracetomol. Or bad migraines due to a violent reaction to an earlier vaccination (vaccinations seem to really upset the immune system and sooner or later, it gets its revenge)!

What the body tries to do, when under siege, is somehow "solve" the intrusive, toxic process. The excretion phase (sneezing, diarrhea, etc.) is only the beginning. If the body cannot rid itself of the active disease toxins, they get deposited in the tissues, to quiet them down.

Cysts are one solution the body uses: a cyst is simply a sac or opening, where the body dumps toxin waste. Fatty (adipose) tissue is another favorite dumping ground of the body. It can get rid of fat-soluble toxins, such as pesticides, solvents etc. The problem is the brain is about 40% fat and it too becomes part of the "trash bin" (dustbin).

Reckeweg produced a famous and persuasive model of this process of deteriorataion, which he called "The 6 Phase Table". The process he called *progressive vicariation* (progressive, in this sense, means getting worse). It starts off mildly enough; but if the process of getting rid of toxins is thwarted, ultimately, cancer could be the price to pay.

NOW you properly understand the term homotoxicology. It is the investigation and removal of auto-toxins, these are self-generated toxins (homo- means self or same) which accumulate within the body and cause damage.

Unlike orthodox medicine (sometimes called allopathic, in contrast), we take the view that it is possible to reverse some of this degeneration process. Wherever you start, you can always improve it, sometimes quite a lot.

WARNING: common sense says that the further down the road of progressive vicariation you go, the harder it is to reverse the process. I've seen homotoxicology remedies work miracles. But you cannot expect to cure everything if there has been a lifetime of abuse and overload.

How Can Homotoxicology Help Against Cancer?

Homotoxicology has a lot to offer in the battle against cancer. I have explained how progressive deterioration of the body's own cleansing system leads to gradual compromise of the defence mechanisms. Eventually, as the process nears an end and the "biological age" of the body tissues (the biological vitality of the tissues, as opposed to the calendar age), neoplasms or cancer changes are seen as almost inevitable on this model.

It makes sense, then, that reversing this process will gain valuable points in the fight against a tumor. The more you help the body recapture its lost biological age, the better it can compete with the invasive cells. It's like turning back the clock!

A basic attack would be to use a detox formula and liver support (there are several), Lymphomyosot, or similar tissue cleanser, and a general anti-viral (more and more cancers are being found to have a viral basis), specific detoxes for acquired vaccine abuse of the immune system (a complex job, requiring skilled medical advice), then tissue stimulants, such as glyoxal and Psorino-heel, and finally, as the situation warrants it, some viscum preparation (mistletoe, a famous anti-cancer herb).

I use HEEL's own Viscum compositum, and alternate it with an Echinacea complex (again, this is a compounded formula, with 25 other ingredients than the Echinacea).

How Can Reckeweg's Cures Help Against Aging?

I have indicated that much of aging in inflammation and "Fire In The Belly" is one of the most devastating aging processes of all.

Homotoxicology helps in two ways. First, it is a better treatment modality. I have already explained that the majority of treatments conventional medicine uses are simply ways of suppressing the disease, not aiding nature in bringing about a cure. Aware doctors have already observed that this simply drives the pathological process underground, only to emerge in later life as a chronic and often degenerative disease.

Homotoxicology not only helps cure the disease, it removes the whole process so that, as it were, there is no mess left behind to haunt the invalid in years to come.

Secondly, there are a number of compounds which will support organs and keep them vibrant and efficient until late in life. Thus there is *Hepar compositum*, to help the liver and *Solidago compositum* or *Populus compositum*, to stimulate kidney drainage. Cerebrum comp. is great for the ageing brain and Ovarium comp. and Testis comp. may help in maintaining the vitality of sex hormones until much later in life. *Aesculus* (horse chestnut) and *Cretaegus* (hawthorn) have been known since times immemorial as cures for arterial and heart problems; now we have *Aesculus comp.* and *Cretaegus-HEEL*.

Homotoxicology Remedies To Beat Inflammation

The classic is *Traumeel*™, one of the greatest remedies in the entire medical repertoire. Sadly, it is only available as a cream or tablets in the USA. The most therapeutically powerful formulation comes in ampoules, for injection, though I and countless others are in the habit of prescribing it in a special oral regime (see below).

The ingredients are:

Botanical ingredients:
- Arnica montana, radix (mountain arnica)
- Calendula officinalis (marigold)
- Hamamelis virginiana (witch hazel)
- Millefolium (milfoil)
- Belladonna (deadly nightshade)
- Aconitum napellus (monkshood)
- Chamomilla (chamomile)
- Symphytum officinale (comfrey)

- Bellis perennis (daisy)
- Echinacea angustifolia (narrow-leafed cone flower)
- Echinacea purpurea (purple cone flower)
- Hypericum perforatum (St. John's wort)

Mineral ingredients:
- Hepar sulphuris calcareum (calcium sulfide)

The exact mechanism of action of TRAUMEEL Injection Solution is not fully understood. Various cellular and biochemical pathways appear to be modulated by the product ingredients. The mechanism of action of TRAUMEEL Injection Solution does not appear to be the result of cyclo-oxygenase or lipoxygenase enzyme inhibition, as is the case with non-steroidal anti-inflammatory drugs (NSAIDs). TRAUMEEL Injection Solution does not inhibit the arachidonic acid pathway of prostaglandin synthesis. Instead, according to data on file with HEEL GmbH, the mechanism of action of TRAUMEEL Injection Solution appears to be the result of modulation of the release of oxygen radicals from activated neutrophils, and inhibition of the release of inflammatory mediators (possibly interleukin-1 from activated macrophages) and neuropeptides.

In vitro studies show that the ingredients in TRAUMEEL Injection Solution are non-cytotoxic to granulocytes, lymphocytes, platelets, and endothelia, which indicates that the defensive functions of these cells are preserved during treatment with TRAUMEEL Injection Solution (Conforti A, et al . Experimental Studies on the Anti-inflammatory Activity of a Homeopathic Preparation. Biomedical Therapy XV No.1:28-31, 1997.).

The anti-inflammatory, anti-edematous, and anti-exudative effects of TRAUMEEL Injection Solution have been demonstrated in clinical trials as well as in vivo experimental models including the carrageenin-induced edema test and the adjuvant arthritis test (ibid.).

Depending on local laws in your country, you may be able to prescribe for yourself. Very many of Reckeweg's remedies are available over the counter and by mail order.

Other formulas to try against inflammation are as follows: *Echinacea comp., Engystol, Lymphomyosot* and *ZEEL* (for inflamed joints).

And for detoxing: *Berberis homaccord, Nux vom homaccord, Lymphomyosot*

You can support important excretion and drainage organs with formulas such as: *Hepar comp* (liver), *Solidago comp* (kidneys), *Populus comp* (kidneys)

Homotoxicology Dosing

All these remedies are best given by injection but all can be taken by mouth, with considerable benefit. You simply place a few drops in water and swallow. They can be mixed together. Some formulations require you dissolve the remedy in a liter or so of water and drink that throughout the day, then skip 2 days and repeat (one day on, two days off, if that's easier)

NOTE: I have used throughout the product names of major German manufacturers HEEL (*herba est ex luce* (Latin): "plants are from light"). I do not get any commissions from them for doing this.

There are other quality producers of complex homeopathy products and we must mention in particular also Dr Reckeweg (company name), Noma and US firms BHI and Deseret Biologicals. Each produces a manual/catalogue which explains the rationale of their formulations in detail.

Best of all in the modern world of homotoxicology could be the Italian firm of *Guna*™.

Websites:

www.heel.com
www.heelusa.com
http://www.cylex-uk.co.uk/company/noma--complex-homoeopathy--ltd-15845329.html
www.gunainternational.com
www.gunainc.com
www.desbio.com

Chapter 14 **Wrap Up**

OK, I've shown you that inflammation is deadly, health-wise. It damages tissues and organs; it makes life painful and unpleasant and measurably shortens our lives. It's bad news.

I've also shown you that around 90% of inflammatory problems start in the gut. That's why I christened it "Fire In The Belly". There is a lot of truth to the old saying "death begins in the colon." I hope I have given you enough understanding to know that you need to get on top of this and stamp out the fires.

I've given you some details of the mechanism of inflammation, including cell responses, chemical responses, and how we measure inflammation, in terms of inflammatory cytokines, c-reactive protein etc.

I listed the major causes of inflammation, starting with inflammatory foods, because they are by far the most important.

But I've also taught you a lot about what has been termed dysbiosis: disordered bowel flora. But we now see disturbances of the balance and make up of organisms in the gut as a far bigger issue.

Because it has emerged that microbial DNA will affect proteins we produce, and this in turn will influence the way we metabolize things, we now regard the whole DNA composite of ourselves and our gut microbes as a "total organism" picture that we call the human microbiome. Colonizing microbes we now call microbiota.

The microbiome contains trillions of significant DNA fragments that do affect us, even though this is counterintuitive.

I have also shared with you the inflammatory importance of heavy metal toxicity and how the excretion pathway for most toxic metals (lead, mercury, etc.) is via the liver and gut. But that sets up inflammation in the bowel, which leads to "leaky gut" and allows heavy metals to be re-absorbed.

They have to be re-excreted along the same pathways but a vicious cycle is set up, in which the body is depleted of important detox molecules, such as glutathione. The whole process has to be corrected properly, otherwise it will not resolve.

Then we got on to a variety of ways to quench this killer "Fire In The Belly". It starts with sorting out your diet.

Then I shared with you how to correct disorders in the microbiome (gut flora), using probiotics and pre-biotics for success.

Then how to skillfully use a variety of anti-inflammatory nutritionals, including such diverse agents as herb teas, key vitamins and mushroom extracts, to help quench the flames.

I introduced you to what may be a very unfamiliar healing paradigm: electro-acupuncture according to (Reinhold) Voll (EAV), coupled with the herbal arts of "homotoxicology". I used the term "deep tissue cleansing', which aptly sums up the very fundamental undercut nature of this approach to reducing inflammation.

I used lots of examples to show how these kindly and gentle formulas can push out old disease shadows, toxins and residues, which may be contributing to disease and a much deeper level than you ever thought possible.

There is more, much more, to the inflammatory model of aging and disease. But you will certainly have realized, reading this text, that it's a vast subject, very complex and changing swiftly. The details are hardly the territory for the lay man or woman.

I've done my best to boil it down to the basics, so that you can understand it and benefit from using what I have explained here.

Sleep

I didn't even mention sleep. But it's a known anti-inflammatory! While you rest or sleep, the body can get on with its repair process.

You need to sleep *in the dark*. Light at night suppresses melatonin, which both reduces inflammation and promotes sleep.

This cuts both ways, meaning that reducing inflammation helps you sleep better. "Fire in the belly" will keep you awake at nights. It also crosses over to "Fire in the brain", remember.

Researchers at UCLA have shown how sleep loss affects the immune system's inflammatory response and suggest sleep interventions as a possible way to address problems associated with inflammation and autoimmune disorders.

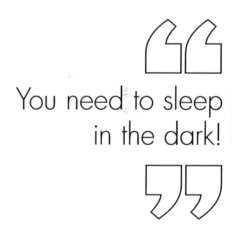

You need to sleep in the dark!

Reporting in the Sept. 6, 2006, edition of the peer-reviewed journal Archives of Internal Medicine, the research team finds that even modest sleep loss triggers cellular and genetic processes involved in the immune system's inflammatory response to disease and injury.

"This study shows that even a modest loss of sleep for a single night increases inflammation, which is a key factor in the onset of cardiovascular disease and autoimmune disorders such as rheumatoid arthritis." said Dr. Michael Irwin, professor and director of the Cousins Center for Psychoneuroimmunology at the Semel Institute for Neuroscience and Human Behavior at UCLA.

Obstructive sleep apnea syndrome, or simply sleep apnea, is a disease process caused by repeated episodes of closing of the upper airway during sleep, resulting in the reduction of airflow and oxygen to the lungs. This can lead to low oxygen levels in the blood stream, gasping episodes and frequent night time awakenings.

Most people with obstructive sleep apnea snore loudly, stop breathing during sleep, and have episodes of gasping, choking, gagging and coughing. Often, the person isn't aware that he is waking up dozens of times during the night as a result of trouble breathing, but these episodes lead to restless sleep and therefore daytime fatigue, regardless of how many hours the person tries to sleep.

Studies suggest that sleep apnea increases inflammation throughout the body (including the lungs). Sleep apnea may cause an increase in inflammatory cytokines. These inflammatory chemicals also contribute to weight gain and obesity, but then we come round in a circle, because obesity is a major cause of sleep apnea.

You know what you need to do. Just do it!

Humor

Those who have read *The Anatomy Of An Illness* by Norman Cousins will also strongly suspect that laughter has powerful anti-inflammatory benefits, probably because of the endorphins it releases.

The notion that psychosocial and societal considerations have a role in maintaining health and preventing disease became crystallized as a result of the experiences of a layman, Norman Cousins. In the 1970s, Cousins, then a writer and magazine editor of the popular Saturday Review, was diagnosed with an autoimmune disease.

He theorized that if stress could worsen his condition, as some evidence suggested at the time, then positive emotions could improve his health. As a result, he prescribed himself, with the approval of his doctor, a regimen of humorous videos and shows like Candid Camera©.

Ultimately, the disease went into remission and Cousins wrote a paper that was published in the New England Journal of Medicine and a book about his experience, Anatomy of an Illness: A Patient's Perspective, which was published in 1979.

The book which resulted in becoming a best seller and led to the investigation of a new field, known then as whole-person care or integrative medicine and now, lifestyle medicine.

Further Particulars

The unscientific foundation that was laid down by Cousins was taken up by many medical researchers including the academic medical researcher Dr. Lee Berk in the 1980s. In earlier work, Berk and his colleagues discovered that the anticipation of "mirthful laughter" had surprising and significant effects. Two hormones – beta-endorphins (the family of chemicals that elevates mood state) and human growth hormone (HGH; which helps with optimizing immunity) – increased by 27% and 87 % respectively in study subjects who anticipated watching a humorous video. There was no such increase among the control group who did not anticipate watching the humorous film.

In another study, they found that the same anticipation of mirthful laughter reduced the levels of three detrimental stress hormones. Cortisol (termed "the steroid stress hormone"), epinephrine (also known as adrenaline) and dopac, (the major catabolite of dopamine), were reduced 39, 70 and 38%, respectively (statistically significant compared to the control group). Chronically released high levels of these stress hormones can be detremential to the immune system.

Lee Berk, DrPH, MPH, a preventive care specialist and psychoneuroimmunologist, of Loma Linda University, Loma Linda, CA, has paired with Stanley Tan, MD, PhD an endocrinologist and diabetes specialist at Oak Crest Health Research Institute, Loma Linda, CA, to examine the effect of "mirthful laughter" on individuals with diabetes. Diabetes is a metabolic syndrome characterized by the risk of heart attack, blindness and other neurological, immune and blood vessel complications. They found that mirthful laughter, as a preventive adjunct therapy in diabetes care, raised good cholesterol and lowered inflammation.

The researchers presented their findings entitled *Mirthful Laughter, As Adjunct Therapy in Diabetic Care, Increases HDL Cholesterol and Attenuates Inflammatory Cytokines and hs-CRP and Possible CVD Risk* at the 122nd Annual Meeting of the American Physiological Society, which is part of the Experimental Biology 2009 scientific conference, April 18-22, 2009, held in New Orleans.

The Study Details

A group of 20 high-risk diabetic patients with hypertension and hyperlipidemia were divided into two groups: Group C (control) and Group L (laughter). Both groups were started on standard medications for diabetes (glipizide, TZD, metformin), hypertension (ACE inhibitor or ARB) and hyperlipidemia (statins). The researchers followed both groups for 12 months, testing their blood for the stress hormones epinephrine and norepinephrine; HDL cholesterol; inflammatory cytokines TNF-α IFN-γ and IL-6, which contribute to the acceleration of atherosclerosis and C-reactive proteins (hs-CRP), a marker of inflammation and cardiovascular disease. Group L viewed self-selected humor for 30 minutes in addition to the standard therapies described above.

Results

The patients in the laughter group (Group L) had lower epinephrine and norepinephrine levels by the second month, suggesting lower stress levels. They had increased HDL (good) cholesterol. The laughter group also had lower levels of TNF-α, IFN-γ, IL-6 and hs-CRP levels, indicating lower levels of inflammation.

At the end of one year, the research team saw significant improvement in Group L: HDL cholesterol had risen by 26 percent in Group L (laughter), and only 3 percent in the Group C (control). Harmful C-reactive proteins decreased 66 % in the laughter group vs. 26 percent for the control group.

Conclusion

The study suggests that the addition of an adjunct therapeutic mirthful laughter Rx (a potential modulator of positive mood state) to standard diabetes care may lower stress and inflammatory response and increase "good" cholesterol levels. The authors conclude that mirthful laughter may thus lower the risk of cardiovascular disease associated with diabetes mellitus and metabolic syndrome. Further studies need to be done to expand and elucidate these findings.

In describing himself as a "hardcore medical clinician and scientist," Dr. Berk says, "the best clinicians understand that there is an intrinsic physiological intervention brought about by positive emotions such as mirthful laughter, optimism and hope. Lifestyle choices have a significant impact on health and disease and these are choices which we and the patient exercise control relative to prevention and treatment."

[This entire section from: American Physiological Society (2009, April 17). Laughter Remains Good Medicine. ScienceDaily. Retrieved March 8, 2012, from http://www.sciencedaily.com /releases/2009/04/090417084115.htm]

FIR saunas

Finally, I should slip this in before the end, just for completeness. Far Infrared (FIR) saunas (have been shown to have beneficial anti-inflammatory effects.

Dr. Sasaki Kyuo, M.D. has done extensive research on the therapeutic uses of far infrared therapy. She is the author of "The Scientific Basis and Therapeutic Benefits of Far Infrared Ray Therapy' - which presents the clinical effects of far infrared ray therapy.

Besides cancer, Dr. Kyuo reports continual successful treatments of many other diseases by use of FIR waves - treatments not only by her but also by many other doctors. The list of diseases - documented in her book - includes stress induced chronic diarrhea, abdominal distention, ulcerated large intestines, gastritis, facial numbness, hemorrhoids, shoulder, back, and knee pain, rheumatism, hypertension, diabetes, weight loss, breast and abdominal tumors, low blood pressure, asthma, anemia, burns and scalds, body odor, early onset of baldness, fracture of cervical vertebra, radiation exposure and related diseases.

In other words, all the "usual suspects" of inflammation and more…

FIR has been shown to:
- It improves micro circulation, by exerting strong rotational and vibrational effects at molecular level.
- Enhances the delivery of oxygen and nutrients in the blood cell to the body's soft tissue areas.
- Promotes regeneration and fast healing. It minimizes the time for "necessary" inflammation.
- Increases metabolism between blood and tissue.
- Enhances white blood cell function, thereby increasing immune response and the elimination of foreign pathogens and cellular waste products. This will reduce inflammation.
- Removes accumulated toxins by improving lymph circulation which is often at the cause of inflammatory problems.
- Stimulate the hypothalamus, which controls the production of neurochemicals involved in such biological processes as sleep, mood, pain sensations, and blood pressure.

Sleeping better, as we have already seen, is a good step towards blocking the process of inflammation.

Well, here we are at the end. You now have a ton of information on "Fire In The Belly" and ways to break the damaging cycle of chronic inflammation.

You'll probably need more information and I can add to all that I have written here with the following:
Diet Wise, my book detailing a comprehensive plan to eliminate inflammatory foods.
www.DietWiseBook.com

The Moldy Patient

A book which concentrates on the Candida and yeasts story, with much more detail than I had room for here.

www.yeastdoctorspeaks.com

The Complete Parasites Handbook

I didn't even touch on parasites as a cause of "Fire In The Belly", except in the case of pork whipworms (page 42). But you'll need to know and understand parasites.

Learn more here: www.parasites911.com

Virtual Medicine

If you really want to follow the EAV and homotoxicology story in more detail (and you should), you'll need to get this book:

www.alternative-doctor.com/virtual_medicine.html

That's all!

Good luck and—of course—good health!

Prof.

Appendix

Hidden Constipation

I learned a lot from my patients over the years. One extraordinary report came from a lady in her forties. She was lively and intelligent; a person I would trust to not make up wild stories.

She had gone in for a colonic irrigation and was surprised at what she saw. Most colonic therapists have a short section of transparent pipe in the enema tube, to allow visualization of the fecal matter being retrieved. Apparently this lady saw some food coloring balls that she quite distinctly remembered was a type she used to eat as a child but had never swallowed in nearly 40 years!

The only conclusion was that this material had been inside her colon for decades.

Now "colonic therapists", or whatever they call themselves, are guilty of many wild claims. Most of them don't go beyond the plumbing idea (I mean, if cleaning out your colon makes you feel so much better, why not take care to put different foods in at the top end? Duh!)

Be especially aware of the bentonite scam that many pull. They get you to swallow bentonite for several days before your appointment and then, presto!... he or she is able to produce skeins of stringy, tarry looking substance from the enema. They claim this is "impacted feces" but in fact it's just the bentonite. That's how it looks when it has passed through the digestive system.

But maybe some of this colonic folk lore is real and has scientific support?

A Danish scientific paper, from researchers at the Gastroenterological Clinic, Elsinore Hospital, put a respectable skin on the topic of long-impacted feces. During a careful and non-sensational enquiry, they found impacted feces or, as they termed it, "hidden constipation", was very real. What's more it was associated with bloating, pain, irregular bowel, diverticula, polyps, hemorrhoids and even malignancy.

So it needs to be taken seriously.

All together, a sample of 251 patients, 159 of them female, was drawn from 645 referred patients, between 1988 and 1999. Nineteen selected symptoms were recorded; plus abdominal palpation, barium enemas and proctoscopy were performed, with special reference to identifying fecal reservoirs.

64% of patients had bloating; 60% abdominal pressure; 26% pain; 58% were tender over the right lower abdomen; 42% had fecal masses and 33% had meteorism (accumulation of gas that makes the abdomen sound like a drum when tapped). None of this was related to age.

But older patients had a much higher incidence of hemorrhoids (grade 2 or more) and diverticula.

62% of patients had detectable fecal mass on the left side; but over 50% also had a *right sided palpable abdominal mass* (additional fecal reservoir).

A malignant tumor was found in four patients, polyps in 20 patients, and in 105 patients left sided diverticula were present.

After a cleansing regimen was conducted the dominant symptoms and signs were reduced significantly. So the colonic therapists are on to a good thing, it seems!

[Dan Med Bull. 2004 Nov;51(4):422-5]

Treatment For Impacted Feces

The Danish researchers used what they called "propulsion therapy" to correct the problems they encountered. We would call it colon cleansing.

There are many products to address this problem. I especially recommend a colon cleanse called *Natural Balance* from my friend Graeme Dinnen (www.resourcesforlife.net)

The following regimen works well for most people, although it may have to be adjusted to suit your particular needs. Finding the correct dosage is important for you to get the best results. Much depends on your condition: those prone to diarrhea or loose stools might react more immediately to the herbs and may find it helpful to start with half a capsule of *Natural Balance* each day; those prone to constipation may need to increase the number of capsules until bowel movements come daily.

Begin with one capsule of *Natural Balance*. The herbs can be swallowed as capsules or made into a herbal tea with warm-hot, rather than boiling water. *Natural Balance* should be taken at night one hour (or more) after supper. Stir the tea to prevent the herbs clumping. The advantage of taking it as a tea is that water helps comfortable detoxification and you are encouraged to drink at least six 8oz. glasses of pure (not distilled) water every day.

Anyone with a chemical sensitivity should start with smaller doses of *Natural Balance* - for example1/4 or 1/2 a capsule a day and contact us for further guidance.

The goal is to have at least 2 bowel movements each day. With *Natural Balance*, if there is no increase in the number of bowel movements within the first three or four days, increase the dosage to two or even three capsules. These can be taken all together. Do not exceed these levels without contacting guidance.

Continue for as long as you feel you are benefitting. This is a gentle yet purgative long-term program which should be taken daily. Although some people have experienced immediate results do not expect them within the first few days. Be ready to honor any bowel movements quickly as your body becomes used to *Natural Balance*. Don't get caught out!

Other Formulas

There are many other formulas in this niche. For example, *Internal Cleansing Fiber* from Ryan Alarid at UltimateLifespan.com here in Las Vegas.

Wherever you shop, look for ingredients like psyllium husk, flax seeds, fennel seeds, licorice root, slippery elm bark, marshmallow root, alfalfa, uva ursi leaf, rhubarb root, peppermint leaves, black seed, cumin seed, cinnamon and ginger root.

There will be other ingredients that people swear by. Try a few formulas!

Plus, of course, you can consider colonic irrigation (deep enemas). Just don't get hooked on the kinky side and remember, what you put in your gut at the top end is far more important than messing around with the output at the other end.

It's still about fire in the belly, but this is maybe the ash pit!

Food Families

Food families we eat. Remember, there is often (but not always) cross-reactivity among members of the same family. If you react to one, do not abandon all other members of that family. But be sure to treat them with care and check whether you are intolerant.

The Plant Kingdom

Apple family: apple, pear, quince, medlar

Avocado family: avocado, cinnamon, sassafras

Banana family: banana, arrowroot, plantain

Beechnut family: beechnut, chestnut

Black pepper

Blueberry family: blueberry (various names), cranberry, wintergreen

Buckwheat family: buckwheat, rhubarb

Carrot family: carrot, celery, parsnip, parsley, dill, fennel, anise, caraway, cumin, coriander

Cashew family: cashew, pistachio, mango

Chicle

Chinese artichoke

Citrus family: orange, grapefruit, lemon, lime, tangerine, citron, kumquat, clementine, ugli

Coffee

Cola family: chocolate, cola, gum karaya

Composite family: lettuce, endive, chicory, globe artichoke, jerusalem artichoke, sunflower, dandelion, chamomile, goldenrod, safflower

Crucifer family: cabbage, brussels sprouts, broccoli, cauliflower, kale, collards, kohlrabi, mustard, turnip, rutabaga, swede, rape, horseradish, chinese leaves, cress

Elderberry

Ginger family: ginger, turmeric

Ginseng

Gooseberry family (saxifrages): gooseberry, blackcurrant, red currant Grape family: grape, muscatel, raisins,sultanas (note: 'currants' are dried grapes)

Grass family: bamboo, barley, wheat, rye, oats, rice, millet, sugar cane, sorghum, corn

Guava family: guava, allspice, clove Gum acacia

Lily family: garlic, onion, shallot, leek, chives, asparagus

Lychee nut

Macadamia nut

Maple sugar

Mint family: peppermint, spearmint, horse mint, water mint, basil, lavender oil, rosemary, marjoram, sage, horehound, savory, thyme

Mulbery family: mulberry, figs, breadfruit

Mushrooms, fungi

Nightshade family: tomato, potato, eggplant, tobacco, green and red peppers, capsicum

Nutmeg family: nutmeg, mace

Okra family: okra (bindi), cottonseed

Palm family: coconut, sago, date, Taro, poi

Papaya

Persimmon

Pineapple

Plum family: plum, prune, peach, apricot, almond, cherry, greengage

Pulses (legumes) family: peanut, pea, beans, lentils, licorice, gum tragancanth, quinoa, sarsaparilla

Spinach family: spinach, chard, beetroot, sugar beet

Squashes family: melon, watermelon, pumpkin, squash, cucumber, courgette, marrow

Strawberry family: strawberry, raspberry, blackberry

Sweet potato

Tapioca

Tea

Vanilla

Walnut family: walnut, pecan, hickory

Water chestnuts

The Animal Kingdom

Sea Food

Anchovy

Bass, mullet, grouper

Butterfish

Carp

Catfish

Cetaceae: whale, dolphin (these are, of course, mammals)

Cod, haddock, hake, coley, whiting

Conger eel

Crustaceae: shrimp, lobster, crayfish, crab

Eel

Fish (there are many families here, apart from the ones already mentioned. Only the

main fishes and groups are included):

Sturgeons

Flounder, turbot, halibut, plaice, dab, sole

Grunt

Herring, pilchards, sprats, shad

Mackerel, tuna, bonito

Pike

Puffer

Red snapper

Salmon, trout

Yellow perch, walleye pike

Molluscs: (Pelecypods) clam, oyster, mussel, scallop; (Gastropods) snail, conch, abalone; (Cephalopods) squid, octopus

Amphibia

Frog

Reptiles

Turtle, snake, alligator

Birds

Duck family: duck, goose

Eggs: all pretty similar, but experiment. Egg white is usually the most allergenic

Grouse family: grouse, turkey, guinea fowl

Pheasant family: chicken, pheasant, quail, partridge, prairie chicken, peafowl Pigeon

Snipe, woodcock

Horse

Lion, tiger

Mammals

Pig: pork, ham, bacon, gammon

Cattle: cow, sheep, lamb,
mutton, goat, buffalo

Rabbit family: rabbit, hare

Rodents: domestic guinea pig

Deer: venison, elk, moose,
caribou, reindeer

Seal

More On The Aspirin Story

On page 71 I reported trials showing that aspirin (salicylic acid) has a surprising protective effect against colo-rectal and other cancers.

Since then, there have been others:

A study just last year (2011) showed taking aspirin significantly reduced the risk of colorectal cancer. 434 subjects taking just a placebo had an incidence of 30 cancers; 427 subjects taking aspirin daily for at least 2 years had an incidence of only 18 cancers.

That's a remarkable 40% reduction. No fancy expensive drugs can do that, or even come close!

The trouble is, as you know, that aspirin has its problems: it causes intestinal bleeding and ulceration.

But now a "new aspirin" gets round that problem.

Here goes the science: the gut lining protects itself from damage ("Fire in the Belly") by secreting nitric oxide (NO) and hydrogen sulfide (HS, stinking rotten eggs gas!) So now Khosrow Kashfi and a team at The City College of New York has developed "NOSH aspirin", a variant that releases its own NO and SH, so protecting the gut to some degree from the ravages of aspirin.

Great—but does it still knock out cancer? Yup!

Kashfi's team tested their NOSH aspirin against 11 human cell lines, including colon, breast, lung, prostate and deadly pancreas cancer.

It was not as good as aspirin alone: **it was 100,000 more potent!** With colon cancer, for example, it caused cancer cells to stop dividing, to wither and die.

Nobody knows yet why NOSH aspirin should have such potent anti-cancer properties. But the good news is that it suggests a far lower—and therefore non-toxic dose of aspirin—would suffice, thus preserving the gut living.

It's very non-toxic in any case. In mice transplanted with human colon cancer, they were fed daily doses of NOSH aspirin sufficient to reduce the tumor size by 85%, yet there was no sign of gut damage.

We could be looking at a human trial within 2 years. This is exciting. Who would have thought it; humble aspirin?

[SOURCE: http://pubs.acs.org/doi/abs/10.1021/ml300002m]

Proof From Up To Date Science

Now a brand new study (April 2012) confirms everything I said in chapter 5 "Our Forgotten Organ" about why inflammatory human microbes in the gut MUST be suppressed and replaced with healthy organisms of the kind we need. A healthy immune system and our very lives depend on it!

Recent research has shed light on the crucial "conversation" between gut microbes and infant genes that appear to help the breast-fed infant make a safe transition from life in the womb to life outside. The study was published April 29, 2012, in the open-access journal Genome Biology reports.

This confirms earlier findings that show breast-feeding gooses the developing immune system. It elucidated the chemical chatter between genes in the developing infants and their gut bacteria by comparing the bacterial communities and genes found in the guts of breast-fed vs. formula-fed (cow's milk) 3-month-olds.

The researchers studied the gut microbiome information and gene expression levels in the infant gut; they identified genes involved in immunity and defense with altered expression levels in relation to the gut bacteria in breast-fed infants.

Breast-fed babies, it emerged, had more diverse gut biota, but their immune systems were ready primed for it. This was almost paradoxical. The babies' fecal matter had more of the obnoxious, virulent organisms (including resistance to antibiotics and toxic compounds), yet the infant immune system was primed and ready to shoot!

What seems to happen is that killer defence genes are activated in the young immune system by the challenge of meeting hostile pathogens.

So it is, in a way, confirmation of the so-called "hygiene hypothesis: if you stay too clean and try to hide from germs, they will get you, because your immune system is compromised from the get-go. Our human microbiome actually EDUCATES the immune system.

The key part, though, is the finding suggesting that human milk promotes the beneficial crosstalk between the immune system and microbe population in the gut, and so maintains intestinal stability.

It's yet another reason not to give kids that garbage from cows, raw or sterilized. Dump that raw milk pansy story, once and for all. It has no relevance or benefit to human development and weakens the immune defences.

Breast is best!

The study was funded by the National Institutes of Health, the Hatch Project Division of Nutritional Sciences Vision, and the United States Department of Agriculture – National Institute of Food and Agriculture (USDA–NIFA) Grant Designing Foods for Health. One author is supported by the College of Arts and Science at Miami University. The authors have disclosed no relevant financial relationships.

[Genome Biol. Published online April 30, 2012. Abstract]

Made in the USA
San Bernardino, CA
16 September 2016